For the established healer or student of the spiritual, this book is enlightening. It permits scientific knowledge and ancient wisdom to meet and be compatible. There are very clear instructions as to the practice of healing with people, animals and places. It clears a path for those wishing to practise the healing arts.

For energy healers wishing to expand their knowledge and understanding it is an invaluable companion, whether to explore the mysteries of energy healing or as a reference book.

For Western medical practitioners willing to open their minds and hearts to energy healing, the book will guide them along familiar paths, showing the connections between their own knowledge and the ancient arts and wisdoms.

Ian Scott,
Fellow of the National Federation of Spiritual Healers

Christina Mark has worked in healthcare for over 40 years. She is trained as a general nurse and a tutor in further education. She is a healing practitioner and tutor with the National Federation of Spiritual Healers and runs courses, seminars and groups in the Scottish Borders.

ENERGY HEALING

The practical workbook

Christina Mark

WATKINS PUBLISHING
LONDON

Distributed in the United States and Canada by
Sterling Publishing Co., Inc.
387 Park Avenue South, New York, NY 10016-8810

This edition first published in the UK and USA 2009 by
Watkins Publishing, Sixth Floor, Castle House,
75–76 Wells Street, London W1T 3QH

1 3 5 7 9 10 8 6 4 2

Designed and typeset by Jerry Goldie

Printed and bound in Great Britain

Library of Congress Cataloging-in-Publication data available

ISBN: 978-1-905857-80-7

www.watkinspublishing.co.uk

For information about custom editions, special sales, premium and
corporate purchases, please contact Sterling Special Sales
Department at 800-805-5489 or specialsales@sterlingpub.com

To my husband, Paul Finegan,
without whose collaboration this book
would not have been completed.

Acknowledgements

I am very grateful to the following people for their support and advice:

Lesley Wood, who inspired me to write this book; Diana Gretton, who encouraged me into healing practice; Patricia Price, who corrected the first draft in great detail; Mary Sutton, who showed me the relevance of the book in a wider context; Mark Campbell, who edited the first draft of the manuscript; James Lees, who motivated me to learn more about energy; Liz Johnstone who arranged and typed the first draft so well; Linda Cessford who typed the second draft so thoughtfully; Denise Leather who drew the logo of the healing hands; Judith Murray whose illustrations brought the bodies, meridians and chakras so vividly to life; Ian Wright who produced the illustrations of the chakras and to Kath Wright who helped with the charts on food combining and blood types; Jamie Richardson who set the energy tables and matched the copy to the artwork with great patience; Peter Finegan who sharpened the chapter on meridians to a fine point; Kate Mark Trelford who provided great hospitality; Janet Bowers who was such a good listener; Charlotte Kelly who was so determined to find the right publisher for the book; Suresh Ariaratnam, whose editing was so finely tuned to the spirit of the book; Shelagh Boyd whose copy-editing contributed so much to the clarity of the book; Samantha Matthews, who proofread the manuscript with its many amendments; Dr Jean Galbraith who wrote the foreword and deepened my understanding of energy; and finally, to Michael Mann, the publisher who made it happen.

Contents

SECTION 1:
ENERGY

SECTION 2:
HEALTH

Illustrations

Foreword

Throughout the Western world there is increasing public use of complementary medicines together with a clear demand for research, and more understanding of the theories behind the many forms of energy medicine. There is also an ever growing demand for theoretical and practical training of therapists which also carries with it professional accountability. 'Energy healers' are now working more widely as volunteers, or paid employees, within UK NHS hospitals, and hospices.

New knowledge and changes in the understanding of spiritual and energy work within 21st-century Western society mean that many textbooks in current use have, to some degree, become out of date. This book brings new theoretical and practical perspectives, and explores the interface between the wisdom of Chinese traditional medicine, the Vedic system, and most modern teaching offered to energy healers. There are few textbooks for healers that include ancient Chinese understanding. Christina draws on her experiences in this area, as well as her years of experience as a registered nurse, a tutor of spiritual healers with the NFSH, and as a healer working within an NHS hospital setting.

Chinese acupuncture has been practised around the world for millennia, and is one of the first complementary therapies to have acquired government statutory status in the UK. Research has shown it can be effective for pain relief, anaesthesia, and an improved quality of life. Patients receiving spiritual healing in general practice will sometimes describe the release of pain through one of the meridian paths out of a finger or toe. Healers can also experience this energetic effect when working with clients. Those giving and receiving healing treatments now have an opportunity to read and see the relevant energetic pathway. With increasing numbers of doctors taking an interest in the subject, it is sensible that there is wider teaching and understanding of the system.

Science is now giving us exciting explanations of subatomic energy transfer in the field of quantum physics. Computer technology can illustrate the vibrational changes brought about by a variety of complementary therapies, particularly those relating to acupuncture points.

In Western orthodox medicine students are taught to be proactive in their treatments, which might be described as offering a yang process. In contrast 'energy therapists', and particularly healers, are taught that the act of channelling healing energy requires a silent mind, in meditational alpha rhythm, which is essentially a passive yin process. There are few orthodox therapists, like the author, who are prepared to undertake the long journey of graduating from a yang into a yin healing approach, and to subsequently achieve a working balance.

This book includes the generally accepted principles of the subtle energy system, the auric fields, the chakras and the meridians. It offers a basic under-standing of human anatomy, and organ functioning. It demonstrates the relationship of vibratory energy as it comes through the subtle energy system to maintain physical, emotional, and psychological health. Similarly, it shows the pathways of clearance of old stress-related energies from the physical body. Problems of sickness are discussed in energy terms, and some reasons are given why such problems could have occurred.

The author has given a great deal of useful detail on the metaphysical and mental relationship of the chakra and meridian system in relation to the four elements, the humours, the constituents and the various parts of the physical body. This is complex information and the student is not required to absorb all the details, but rather to understand the general principles involved. As the author advises, not every expression may ring true for every reader, we have all travelled different paths.

The author understands the importance of meditation and describes those that she feels to be safe for the modern student. In particular, she understands the difficulties and potential dangers that may result from meditations that attempt to raise energy up the chakras, particularly for those people who have already had negative kundalini experiences. She has therefore only encouraged meditations relating to the opening and closing of chakras from the crown to the base. The reason for this need for change relates to several factors. Amongst these are Western independent multispiritual input, the greater use of drugs, alcohol, and earlier sexual activity among the young since the 1960s, which may destabilize the base chakra, and higher chakras.

As an NFSH healer, Christina understands the importance of unconditional love and humility in the healing process. No healer is truly in conscious control of the energy changes that occur. In the section of her book covering 'the ties that bind' the author offers important exercises for the student to help clear emotional and mental bonds that tie them to outdated ideas, people, and actions. The process of letting go is the beginning of a more profound spiritual process of forgiving, and asking for forgiveness at the deepest, or the highest, level depending on one's belief system. Many of the most fundamental and older blockages may be found in the finer vibratory levels of the soul and spiritual fields of the aura. These blocks usually relate beyond this life to problems of the unconscious past.

The last part of the book relates to practical healing issues, including material for teachers of healing. In addition, there are important sections on kinesiology, distant healing, working with animals, and working in hospices and hospital environments.

Once students discover the importance of energy pathways and their importance to life issues, both known and unknown, then the harbour opens to a vast ocean of knowledge. This book is just a short sail into it. Clearly, standing on its own this book is not enough to teach a student to be a practising healer or any other complementary therapist. It does, however, offer excellent background knowledge integrating Eastern, Far Eastern, and Western knowledge of healing energy. I unreservedly recommend this book to all those who wish to learn more about the processes of energy healing.

Dr Jean Galbraith
Vice Chair, London Branch,
Doctor–Healer Network

Introduction

Some questions and answers on energy, health and healing

This book is designed as a handbook, to guide the reader through the fundamental principles and practices of working with energy.

Energy fuels all of us, yet is unique in its arrangement in everyone because we are all unique in our essential nature. The condition of a person's health is a reflection of how this energy is balanced in the mind, body and soul. Healing is a response to the state of health when energy becomes imbalanced or weakened either through the food we eat, the way we live, the surroundings we inhabit or the interplay amongst them. Healing may take many forms such as medication, surgery or therapeutic touch, but the most ancient and enduring of all these practices is to work directly with energy itself.

This form of healing evolves naturally through the alignment of the mind, body and soul. It is not given to diagnose or to promise a cure as such, but to support energy as it is redirected during the act of healing. Working directly with energy through the power of thought, for energy follows thought, can deepen the understanding of the entire organism, including the aura, the chakras and the meridians, which support the structures and functions of the physical form. This work is guided by energy itself, through the process of grounding, attunement, protection and permission, so that both the practitioner and patient enter into the healing state in a unified field of energy.

The book is an invitation to learn about the language of energy, to explore how it works and to develop the skills which gather together energy, health and healing into a coherent whole.

Can anyone work with healing energy?

Healing energy is a universal gift open to everyone. Developing that gift starts from an interest in healthcare and grows with a willingness to learn about the flow of energy and how it affects health and healing. You have to be prepared to be a good listener, to disengage from your own perspective so that you are able to listen not just to the words, but to what lies behind them, and to the areas where the flow of energy becomes trapped or diverted. You need to be in a reasonable state of health yourself, to be prepared to learn some basic first-aid skills and to share your interest in healing with others. It is necessary to be open to all forms of healthcare, both conventional and complementary, to develop an integrated perspective.

What may I gain from this book personally?

The more you study energy the more you can become aware of its continual exchange happening all around us. Whether we see it or not, this affects each of us and, as we study, the clearer the understanding becomes of the essential interconnectedness of energy everywhere and the ways it can become trapped and blocked. This growing understanding helps insight into the reasons for illnesses and accidents; it encourages the experience of the deeper state of awareness through which healing energy is transmitted and received. It brings with it a growing integration of the state of healing consciousness into other areas of life and helps us not only in making choices and fulfilling our daily obligations, but also in developing a more compassionate relationship with ourselves and with others, so that the reality of healing is ever present.

What may I gain from this book professionally?

You should gain an increasing familiarity with the language of energy as it is expressed in the aura, the chakras, the meridians and the body systems. This is accompanied by an understanding that the physical expression of every patient is a manifestation of what is happening throughout the seven levels of energy in the body. This in turn brings an awareness that the spiritual needs of every patient or client are of fundamental importance to their well-being, whether or not they are aware of them. Such an awareness naturally leads to an acceptance of the unique nature of every patient or client and shows how the specific contents of their treatment are determined.

Further study increases the insights into the different states of mind of every patient, revealing the link between the body and the soul. This helps us to recognize the relevance of energy healing work in all forms of healthcare, as it provides an infinite source of renewable and sustainable energy. Developing awareness of the continual exchange of energy also reveals the importance of protecting personal energy when working in healthcare and in daily life so that it is not depleted by extensive physical or psychological contact.

What is energy healing?

Energy healing works directly with energy itself without any intermediary; it is unconditional in its potential to treat imbalances in body, mind and soul. It is the most ancient and enduring form of healthcare, an instinctive, innate response which can be developed through education in the language of energy and the practice of healing. Energy healing works at every stage of life from conception until death, whatever the circumstances and states of health; it is often strengthened in those who have developed their spiritual perspective. It treats conditions that have been inherited as well as those acquired through life experience.

Energy is directed for healing through the immune system, the body's defence mechanism, which provides protection for both the body and mind. Physical traumas and habitual negative thought patterns act as blockages and restrict the natural flow of healing energy which is generated more effectively when body and mind are in harmony. Such blockages impede the work of the immune system and one of the functions of healing energy is to dissolve them, thus restoring the natural flow of energy throughout the body.

What makes energy healing different from all other forms of healthcare?

Other forms of healthcare use techniques such as medication, surgery or manipulation to produce their results. Energy healing in its most essential form works simply through the power of thought when a request for healing to take place is made by the practitioner on behalf of the patient, when they are united in the presence of the consciousness of healing. It can be accessed instantaneously, whenever and wherever healing energy is required. It works purely through attunement to the energy of healing, whether in the presence of the patient or, indeed, at any distance. Direct contact is not necessary. It works through any or all of the seven levels of energy that may need attention, without any specific guidance from the practitioner. It is the healing energy itself which guides the nature of the treatment.

It can work in harmony both with complementary therapies and medical practices because it can provide the essential healing energy which supports all therapeutic procedures, helping them to work to their maximum effectiveness.

Above all, it is a natural process inherent in all life forms which only becomes limited when energy itself becomes blocked or weakened through any sort of trauma at any level: physical, psychological or spiritual.

Is there any proof that energy healing works?

Energy healing works on the basis that everyone is unique and will, therefore, respond differently to every treatment, according to their specific situations. There are, however, some physical and psychological changes which may be observed or measured before and after healing treatments. These include:

- ◆ adjustment of blood pressure;
- ◆ adjustment in breathing rates;
- ◆ balancing of arterial pulses;
- ◆ relief of pain;
- ◆ more agility in physical movement;
- ◆ improved patterns of sleeping;
- ◆ more peaceful and focused state of mind.

What will this book include?

This book explores the nature of energy and its relationship with health and healing in the following ways:

- ◆ By detailing the circulation of energy through the seven levels which constitute the field of the aura which surrounds every living form.
- ◆ By describing how energy within the body interacts with energy in the external environment.
- ◆ By showing how energy moves into form and how it affects physical, psychological and spiritual health.
- ◆ By demonstrating how energy may be sensed through the processes of grounding, attunement, protection and permission.
- ◆ By exploring the relevance of energy healing throughout the seven stages of life.

◆ By showing how to use energy healing when working with animals, with the land and in buildings.

◆ By clarifying the role of energy healing within professional healthcare.

Section 1

ENERGY

1.1

Connecting with Energy

The aim of this section on energy is *connection*: to establish the link between energy in its outermost form of the aura and its most tangible presence in its physical state, which is the body. This connection binds together the seemingly disparate constitutions of the aura, chakras, elements, meridians, glands, hormones, nerves and the body processes, showing that they are in actuality mirror reflections of one another. Together they manifest the movement of consciousness, the highest expression of energy, through its journey from light into form.

The modern understanding of the relationship between light, in its expression of energy, and form, in its expression as matter, unfolded through the work of Albert Einstein, the scientist and mystic, who formulated the equation $e = mc^2$; where e relates to energy, m to mass, and c to the speed of light. He revealed through mathematical calculation that energy and matter are two expressions of a universal source. Moreover, Einstein showed space and time as being intimately connected, referring to them as a four-dimensional space-time continuum, propelled by electromagnetic and gravitational interactions not fixed in sequence, but witnessed entirely in relation to the eye of the observer, and to the speed of the light of the observations. In other words, everything is in relationship to everything else.

This connection between energy and matter developed further through the work of the quantum physicists, who explored the quantities or packets of energy in atoms, the smallest cellular particles that are capable of being distinguished for a specific function. Although atoms consist of particles called protons and neutrons with a surrounding cloud of electrons, these constituents behave with wave-like properties, and indeed all matter is now considered to exhibit a wave-particle duality that has both fluid and particulate properties. We can see that both electricity and light, for example, demonstrate a wave form characterized as flow, and yet certain properties may only be explained by the existence of consistuent particles – electrons in the case of electricity and photons in the case of light. Energy may be differentiated in many forms – chemical, kinetic, gravitational, thermal, etc. – but also may be converted from one form into another according to circumstances.

This state of affairs reveals itself in the energetic behaviour of all sensate beings:

◆ through the seven layers of the aura, in which colours shift, merge, re-emerge, and rearrange themselves.

◆ through the seven chakras, the wheels of energy which turn at different speeds to circulate energy through the physical body.

◆ through the seven pairs of meridians, the pathways which allow energy to flow to and from all the body systems.

◆ through the seven glands, the ductless organs which provide and secrete hormones into the physical body so that it can make the changes that are required.

◆ through the hormones, the substances that set in motion the changes that are needed in mind and body.

◆ through the nerves, which act as the central control system, the headquarters of communication for mind and body, and which act in conjunction with the glands and the hormones that they release.

◆ through the seven body processes, which incorporate the anatomy and physiology of every living being and through the instantaneous responses which maintain and preserve the being in life.

These processes are all, however, affected by the external environment of their surroundings and by the internal environment of thoughts and feelings. These seven aspects of energy demonstrate the interconnected nature of life. On all levels of energy a similar pattern emerges; of energy which does not disappear but retains its essential components, whilst having the mutability to respond to its surroundings.

Within this function there are two aspects, being and doing. As humans we do what is necessary to maintain our lives. *Being* takes place only in the present moment, where stillness and stability can be found. *Doing*, on the other hand, is a place of action and purpose, and can be located across time. All real relationships are built on an inner stability and an outer flexibility, where nothing is fixed and yet where there is a natural order that appears in creation.

It is energy that provides the fuel for our lives and for the world that we live in. By learning about the flow of energy we will not only learn more about ourselves and the world we live in, but also about the relationship between the two. We can therefore describe the continuous link between energy and being that is fundamental to energy healing as follows:

- In the light of consciousness there is energy.
- In energy there is being.
- In being there is form.
- In form there is action.
- In action there is reaction.
- In reaction there is change.
- In change there is the light of consciousness, to bring it into being.

1.2

Energy through Light into Form

As above, so below.

ANON

Matter is the tangible appearance of energy as it expresses itself in the journey through light into colour, sound and form. There is a continuum of expression of consciousness manifesting itself as the universal source of life which is carried through energy. Given that energy underlies all form it is necessary to explore something of its nature and how it affects our minds and bodies.

Investigating the relationship between the body systems, the meridians, the chakras, the aura, and light itself, reveals the interconnectedness not only of mind and body but also of all life forms, from the smallest creature to the greatest solid mass, from a single cell to the planets of the solar systems.

The seven bodies of energy traditionally are known as the divine, the spirit, the soul, the mind, the astral, the etheric, and finally the physical form of the body. This most beautiful and scientific construction vibrates with energy throughout its lifetime, absorbing and assimilating it from the divine, from the inspiration of the spirit, the nurture of the soul, the stimulus of the mind, and the framework of the etheric body. Energy may become blocked or split but it is never destroyed. It is either reformulated or released, and returns to its universal source to be used endlessly for the expression of life in every form. Energy comes from an infinite source which animates all of creation. It moves cyclically, turning and returning in a sequence that is mirrored throughout the universe, be it the changing of the seasons or the rotation of the planets.

In its outermost and most visible form it equates in the auric field to the colour purple, and is known as the divine body, which is the deepest source of all realized contact. From the purity of the divine it extends into the expression of spirit, which equates with blue, the colour of inspirational thought. Spirit cannot be destroyed. It is in constant movement, animating the chakras. From the spirit it flows into the soul body, which provides a place for it during its sojourn on this plane of existence. The soul body equates with turquoise, the colour of expressive thought, revealing itself in the meridians, which lie just beneath the surface of the skin. Just as the soul is receptive to the spirit by providing it with a setting, so the meridians are receptive to the life force by directing energy through a network of interconnecting pathways into the systems of the physical body.

Energy extends through the soul into the mind body, where consciousness is seated. The mind body equates in the auric field with green, the colour of nature, showing itself through the activity of the autonomic and central nervous systems. These systems activate all the senses, providing the mind with stimuli without which it cannot function. The mind body is the centre point of the seven bodies and all the others may be accessed through it and illuminated by it.

Energy then travels through the mind into the astral body, which represents the emotions. The astral body equates with yellow, the colour of emotional thought, revealing itself in the endocrine system, whose hormones set all the structures and forms into motion. Just as the hormones released by the endocrine system act as a catalyst to the outer form, so the emotions generated from the astral body trigger the inner form, the faculties of consciousness, in all the range and depth of their expression. Energy moves through the astral into the etheric body, which provides the template that shapes and guides all the structures and functions of the living form. The etheric body equates with orange, the colour of creative thought, as it reveals itself in the template of the blood. It is the blood that carries the living power of creation, building the conditions for living by transporting the nutrients necessary to make life possible. The etheric body fills all space and supports the propagation of electromagnetic radiation, without which the life force and its nutrients would have no foundation and structure to manifest into the physical body. Finally the energy completes its journey in the physical body, which equates with red. Here is all the potential for expression encompassing the whole spectrum of possibilities from the most uplifting to the most oppressive.

Just as energy can never be fixed neither can human potential in its ability to move forward, to adapt and start anew.

Energy moves through these seven levels continually. In turn the body regenerates energy through breathing, eating and drinking, returning it via the meridians and chakras, so that it encircles the seven levels of energy that constitute the auric field.

With understanding may come an awareness and an appreciation of the underlying intelligence that governs and directs the flow of energy, and which comes into its most potent and comprehensive expression in the human being.

The human being has been given a twofold responsibility: to be receptive to the innate intelligence as it makes itself known through the consciousness of each of us and to act on it according to our individual measure for our well-being. When this comes about there is an ease of flow within the energy field, in which the light of consciousness finds clear expression in the minds and bodies of those willing to respond to it. The study of energy brings light to every level it explores, from the level of the spirit to its most tangible expression in the visible form.

Energy through light into form

Colour	Aura	Chakra	Meridian	Nerve	Hormone	Function
White into Purple	Divine	Crown	Governor vessel Bladder & kidney Gall bladder & liver	Cerebral cortex	Cerebral, e.g. melatonin	Sensation
Blue	Spirit	Brow	Governor vessel Stomach & spleen Bladder & kidney Gall bladder & liver	Hypothalamus	Hypothalamic, e.g. pituitrin	Adaptation
Turquoise	Soul	Throat	Governor & conception vessels Large Intestine & lung Stomach & spleen Bladder & kidney Triple Heater & heart protector	Cervical Ganglia Medulla	Respiratory, e.g. thyroxine	Respiration
Green	Mind	Heart	Governor & conception vessels Lung & large intestine Spleen & stomach Heart & small Intestine Kidney & bladder Triple heater & heart protector Gall bladder & Liver	Cardiac plexus	Cardiac, e.g. thymosin	Circulation
Yellow	Astral	Solar plexus	Governor & conception vessels Stomach & spleen Kidney & bladder Liver & gall bladder	Solar plexus	Digestive, e.g. Insulin; glycogen	Digestion
Orange	Etheric	Sacral	Governor & conception vessels Spleen & stomach Kidney & bladder Liver & gall bladder	Sacral plexus	Reproductive, e.g. oestrogen; progesterone; testosterone	Regulation
Red	Physical	Base	Governor & conception vessels Spleen & stomach Kidney & bladder Liver & gall bladder	Coccygeal	Articular, e.g. adrenaline; cortisone	Articulation

1.3

Energy through Form into Body

For of the soul the body form doth take;
For soul is form, and doth the body make.

EDMUND SPENSER, *HYMN IN HONOUR OF BEAUTY*

The physical body processes energy through a series of interconnected systems that keep it in working order. The balanced relationship between each system and all of its parts is maintained by the flow of the energy that holds and sustains every living form. The greater the understanding and appreciation of the movement of this energy throughout the seven body processes, the more able we are to make informed choices regarding our health, and also to nurture ourselves. The physical body is the most tangible and articulate expression of energy; because it is visible and accessible it acts as a gateway, inviting us to explore more deeply the other six levels of energy.

It is fundamental for anyone who wishes to take an active responsibility for their own health, and for anyone who is working with energy in any capacity, either in conventional or complementary therapies, to learn about the core functions of the seven body processes. Learning about the anatomy and physiology of the body provides a framework for the understanding of the more subtle and less visible levels of influence which are operating within the organism and which contribute to a more comprehensive understanding of the links between physical, psychological and spiritual health.

The Seven Body Processes

Articulation: for structure and movement in the skeleton, muscles and joints.

Regulation: for balance and renewal in the kidneys and the sexual organs.

Digestion: for nourishment and evacuation in the stomach, spleen, pancreas, gall bladder, liver, and small and large intestine.

Circulation: for transportation and protection in the heart, blood and lymph vessels.

Respiration: for inhalation and exhalation in the lungs.

Adaptation: for reaction and adjustment through the hormones.

Sensation: for perception and response through the central and autonomous nervous systems.

Articulation

The articular process enables physical movement to take place by providing a construction in flexible sections. It consists of the bones of the skeleton (see figure 1), the joints which act as hinges between them, and the muscles which activate the momentum for movement. This system links the body to the mind so that it can carry out its instructions, and so becomes a construction for consciousness.

Bones consist of 70 per cent minerals (mainly calcium and magnesium) and 30 per cent collagen which is a powerful, elastic protein. The structure of bone is in three layers:

◆ The outer layer is compact and contains blood vessels and lymph vessels.

◆ The middle layer is hollow and contains bone marrow, which produces red and white blood cells.

◆ The inner layer is spongy to allow movement to take place.

Figure 1: Energy through the skeleton

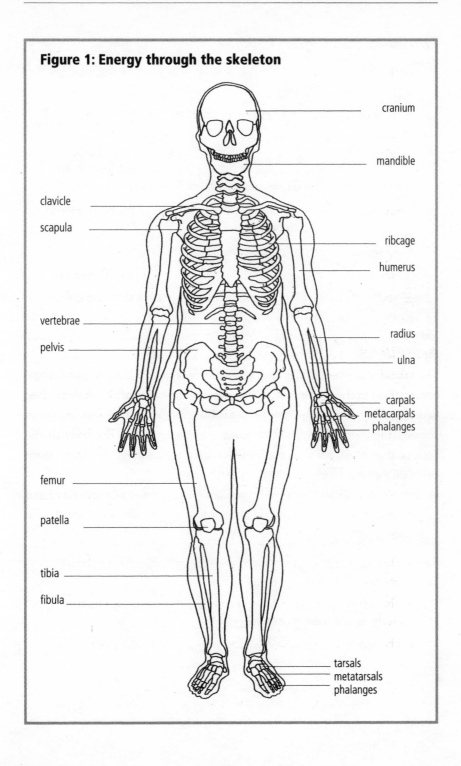

cranium

mandible

clavicle

scapula

ribcage

humerus

vertebrae

pelvis

radius

ulna

carpals
metacarpals
phalanges

femur

patella

tibia

fibula

tarsals
metatarsals
phalanges

Functions of the skeleton

The skeleton:

- gives shape to the body;
- holds the body upright;
- protects the inner organs;
- enables the body to move with the aid of the muscles (see figure 2);
- enables the body to bend with the aid of the joints;
- stores minerals;
- makes blood cells;
- enables cutting, tearing, crushing, grinding in the form of teeth.

There are over 1,000 muscles in the body composed of groups of elastic fibres gathered together in bundles, bound by a thick band and enclosed in a sheath. Skeletal muscles are attached to bones by tendons and have two points of attachment – the point of origin where the muscle remains relatively fixed, thus preventing movement from taking place during the contraction of the muscle; and the point of insertion where the muscle becomes flexible, thus allowing movement to take place during contraction. Muscles receive stimuli from motor nerves, and respond by contracting; they usually work in pairs so that one acts – the synergist, and the other one reacts – the antagonist. The relationship between the two creates muscle tension.

Muscles can be divided into two categories according to their function:

TYPES OF MUSCLE

VOLUNTARY	INVOLUNTARY
Controlled by the nervous system	Controlled by the autonomic nervous system
Work on request	Work automatically
Control movements outside the body	Control movements inside the body
Maintain the skeleton	Maintain the inner organs
Work in pairs	
Attached to bones by tendons	

Figure 2: Energy through muscles

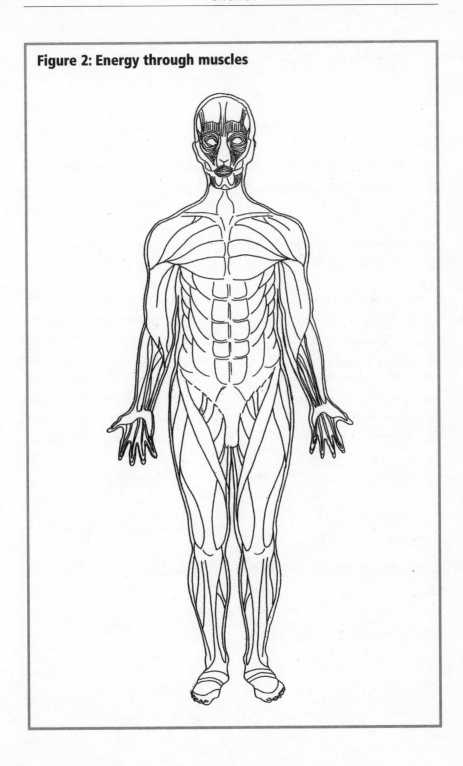

Joints are places where bones or cartilage meet. There are three types of joint structure: cartilginous, fibrous and synovial (see figure 3).

Cartilaginous

These joints are covered with cartilage, enclosed in a fibrous capsule and have some movement. They are found between the ends and the shaft of long bones in growing children, between the first rib and the top of the sternum, and in the sacroiliac joints in the pelvis.

Fibrous

Fibrous joints are held together with collagen and exhibit minimal movement. They are found in the skull and in the teeth.

Synovial

These joints are filled with synovial fluid and exhibit flexible movement. They are found in all freely moveable joints. Synovial joints are classified in four groups according to the range of movements of the bones. They act as hinges to the bones and are held in place by ligaments. Movement is lubricated with synovial fluid and cushioned by cartilage.

Ball and socket: circular range of movement, e.g. in the hip and shoulder setting.

Hinge: movement in one direction only, e.g. in fingers, toes, elbows and knee setting.

Gliding: gliding movement both side to side and back and forth are restricted, e.g. in the carpal bones of the wrist setting.

Saddle: wide range of movement side to side and back and forth, e.g. in the thumb setting.

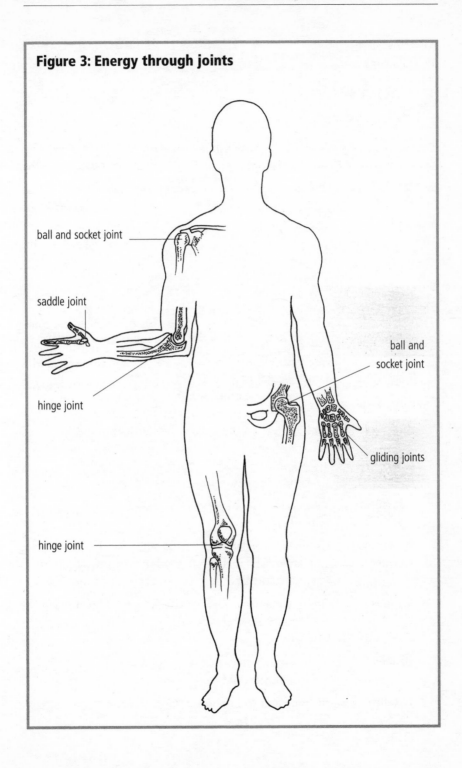

Figure 3: Energy through joints

ball and socket joint

saddle joint

ball and
socket joint

hinge joint

gliding joints

hinge joint

Regulation

The regulation process operates in two ways through:

◆ the urinary function, and

◆ the reproductive function.

The reproductive systems work in conjunction with the kidneys and the adrenal glands to bring about life. Blood is cleansed and purified by the kidneys so that life can be maintained. Adrenaline is produced by the adrenal glands, which rest on the top of each kidney, so that life can be renewed. In safeguarding the functions and structures of the body, the regulation system becomes the guardian of consciousness.

The Urinary System

The components of the urinary system (see figure 4) are as follows:

Kidneys:	located in the small of the back, kidneys filter all the blood in the body every 7–14 minutes.
Nephrons:	long tubes located in the kidneys, closed at one end and open at the other, leading into a cluster of tiny blood vessels known as the glomeruli. Act as the filtering units of the kidneys, by purifying the blood and transforming waste fluids into urine. Some water and valuable substances in the blood are reabsorbed back into the body through the long tubules.
Glomeruli:	the cup-like end of the nephrons containing the minute blood vessels.
Bowman's capsule:	the network of capillaries at the end of each glomerulus which allows most of the filtering of the blood to take place. Filtered fluid becomes urine.
Ureters:	two fine muscular tubes 26–30cm long leading from the kidneys, through which urine passes down into the bladder.
Bladder:	an elastic muscular sac which holds urine – 700–800ml of urine at a stretch!
Urethra:	the tube that empties the bladder of urine.

Figure 4: Energy through the urinary system

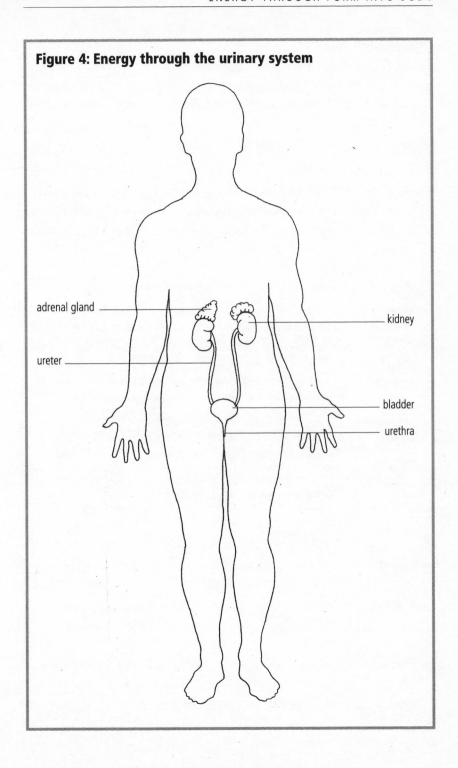

adrenal gland

kidney

ureter

bladder

urethra

Female Reproduction

The system develops at puberty, through the action of the pituitary gland. The hormones secreted are oestrogen and progesterone, which are responsible for the development of female genitals, the growth of underarm and pubic hair, development of breasts, onset and control of menstrual cycle and the maintenance of pregnancy. The components of the female reproductive system (see figure 5), are as follows:

Vagina:	around 10cm/4in long, set at a right angle to the womb and arranged in folds, this muscular channel runs from the neck of the womb to the exterior of the body. It accommodates the penis and acts as the birth canal for a baby.
Cervix:	the neck of the womb, linking the uterus to the vagina.
Uterus:	hollow organ with very powerful muscles and lined with endometrium. Monthly menstruation is the release of lining of the womb and unfertilized egg. Receives the fertilized egg and protects and nourishes the developing foetus until birth.
Fallopian tubes:	fine tubes down which the egg travels from the ovary to the uterus. Conception takes place in the Fallopian tubes before the egg reaches the uterus.
Ovaries:	these organs secrete oestrogen and progesterone, and produce eggs ready for fertilization.

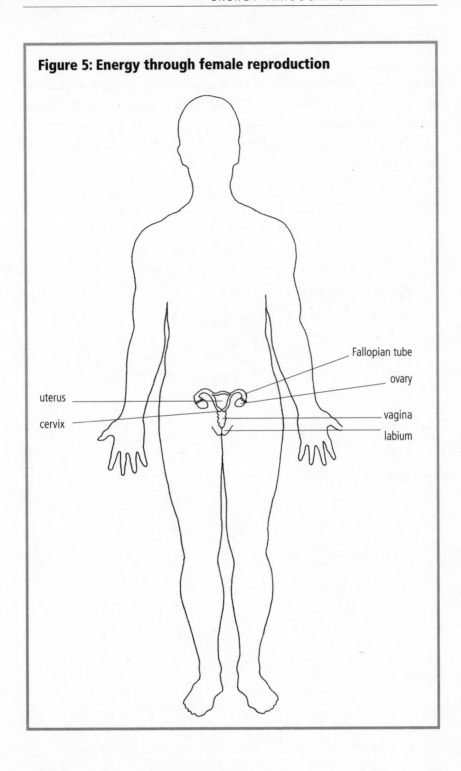

Figure 5: Energy through female reproduction

Male Reproduction

The system develops at puberty when the hormone testosterone is released, which is responsible for the development of male genitals, growth of facial and body hair, deepening of the voice and developing the male physique. Each day the adult male may produce 300 million sperm – although it takes only one sperm to fertilize an egg, it is improbable that this will happen unless over 200 million sperm are produced.

The components of the male reproductive system (see figure 6) are as follows:

Penis: for passing urine and sperm.

Testes: for producing testosterone and making sperm – 10–30 million sperm cells form in the testes every month.

Epididymis: where sperm mature.

Vas deferens: the tubes connecting the internal and external organs (penis and testes).

Seminal vesicles: for storing sperm and producing semen supported by the prostate gland and the bulbourethral glands.

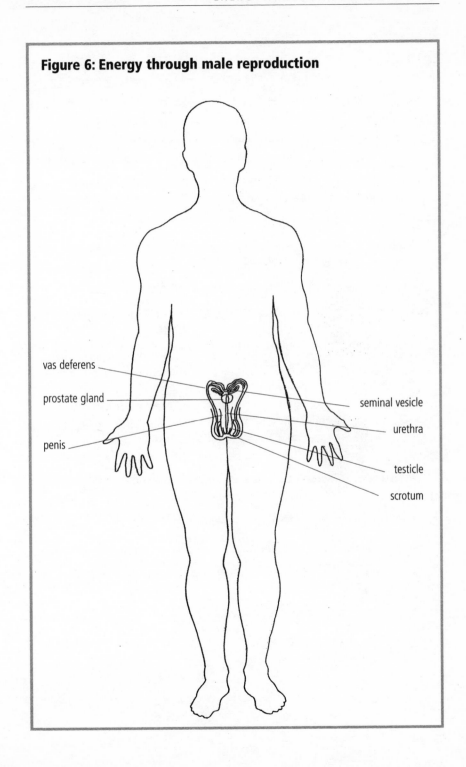

Figure 6: Energy through male reproduction

vas deferens

prostate gland

penis

seminal vesicle

urethra

testicle

scrotum

Digestion

The digestive process takes place through one long tube, which begins in the mouth and ends at the anus. (It is said that if you laid your intestines out in a straight line, they would be nearly six times as long as your height.) With this process, the body ingests food, assimilates nutrients that it can work with, stores substances that it cannot utilize immediately, and clears away the waste products to the best of its ability. This process becomes the harvest for consciousness because it is given the fuel it requires to nurture its expression.

Food is propelled through the digestive system by a sequence of muscular contractions known as peristalsis. The journey for food has five stages:

Mouth: Food is softened in the mouth by chewing it into a pulp with the help of saliva.

Oesophagus: (or gullet) transports food into the stomach.

Stomach: holds food for about four hours. Breaks down some proteins into amino acids, digests milk, some medications and alcohol. Passes its contents into the small intestine.

Small intestine: this is about six metres long. Breaks down proteins into amino acids, carbohydrates into monosaccharides and fats into fatty acids and glycerol, into molecules small enough to be absorbed into the blood.

Large intestine: this is about three metres long. Takes the food substances which cannot be broken down and releases them as faeces through the anus.

Other organs involved in digestion and excretion are:

◆ the pancreas, which produces insulin to change sugars into glucose,

◆ the gall bladder, which stores bile to break down and concentrate fats and oils,

◆ the liver, which processes digested food.

See figure 7 for an illustration of the components of the digestive system.

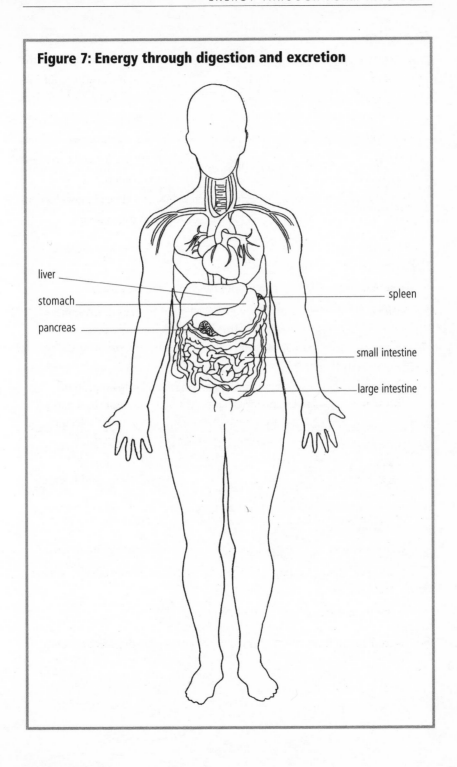

Figure 7: Energy through digestion and excretion

liver

stomach

pancreas

spleen

small intestine

large intestine

Circulation

The circulatory system consists of:

- the heart, which pumps blood around the body;
- the blood vessels, through which red blood cells are pumped; and
- the lymph glands, through which white blood cells are pumped.

The circulatory process supplies the ingredients to sustain the life force. In this way it becomes the dynamo for consciousness, carrying all that is required to maintain and preserve the physical form for its duration in this life (see figures 8, 9, 10 and 11).

The Heart

The heart (see figure 8) is a pump (about the size of your fist), made of smooth, striated muscle and protected by the pericardium, a sac of watery fluid which surrounds it. The heart contains four chambers that form two separate networks. The upper chambers, the atria, receive blood and the lower chambers, the ventricles, pump it out. They are separated by the septum, which prevents oxygenated and deoxygenated blood from mixing with one another. The chambers are connected by one-way valves that prevent a back-flow of blood.

The heart beats at around 60–80 beats per minute in an adult. It enables the blood to transport oxygen and nutrients to all parts of the body and to remove carbon dioxide and other waste products from all parts of the body. The systolic pressure of blood measures the strength of the heart beat and the diastolic indicates the pressure between the heart beats. Average blood pressure measurement are as follows:

Baby	90/60mmHg
Adult	120/90mmHg
Elderly	150/80mmHg

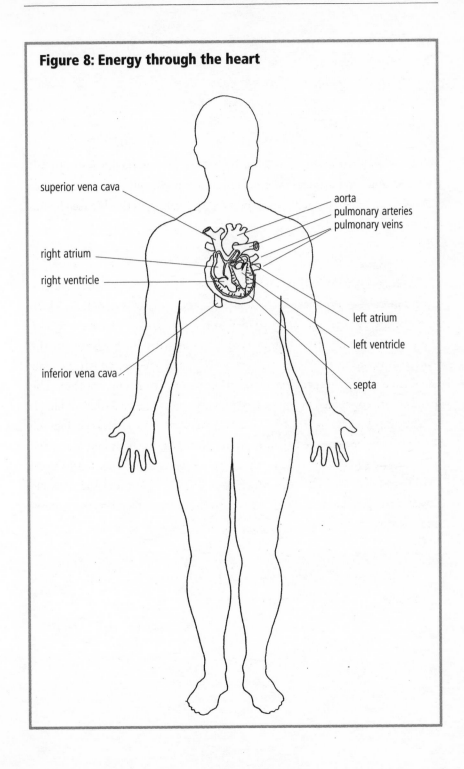

Figure 8: Energy through the heart

superior vena cava

aorta
pulmonary arteries
pulmonary veins

right atrium

right ventricle

left atrium

left ventricle

inferior vena cava

septa

The Arteries

The French have a saying : 'You are only as young as your arteries.'

Artery walls are thick and are surrounded by muscle to sustain the pressure of the blood being pumped through them. Arterial blood has a pulse in its flow and is bright red. Arteries transport blood containing oxygen in a spiralling force of energy; the oxygenated blood travels from the lungs to the heart and passes through the left side of the heart to the rest of the body in a figure-of-eight pattern. Arterial blood also carries:

- ◆ nutrients to contribute to the generation of energy;
- ◆ water to maintain the hydration of the body;
- ◆ red blood cells to carry oxygen;
- ◆ white blood cells to fight infection;
- ◆ enzymes to act as catalysts for change; and
- ◆ hormones to make the changes happen.

Arteries divide into narrower tubes called arterioles, which subdivide into a mesh of capillaries, through which oxygen diffuses out and carbon dioxide diffuses in. The capillaries are then drawn together to form venules, which join with one another to become veins, which return de-oxygenated blood to the heart.

Figure 9 shows the arrangement of the major arteries in the body.

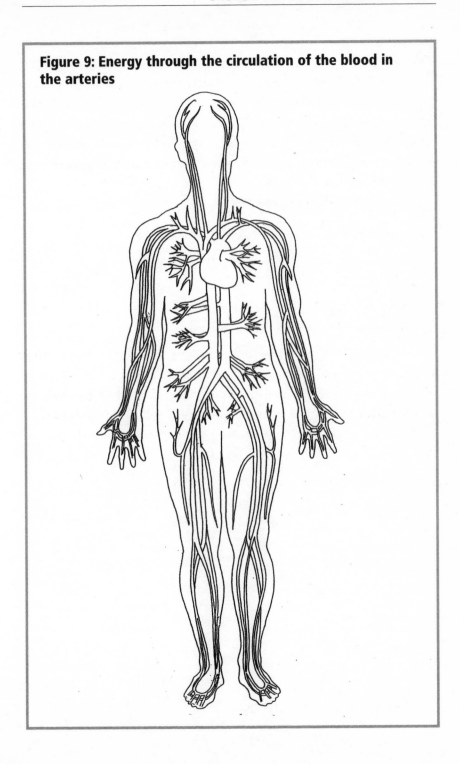

Figure 9: Energy through the circulation of the blood in the arteries

The Veins

If you are only as young as your arteries then you are only as old as your veins.

Vein walls are thin and less elastic than artery walls because blood is pumped through them under less pressure. Veins have valves to prevent a backflow of blood and vein blood is dark red. Veins transport blood containing carbon dioxide in a spiralling flow of energy; deoxygenated blood returns through the veins into the right side of the heart and back to the lungs in a figure-of-eight pattern.

Figure 10 shows the arrangement of the major veins in the body.

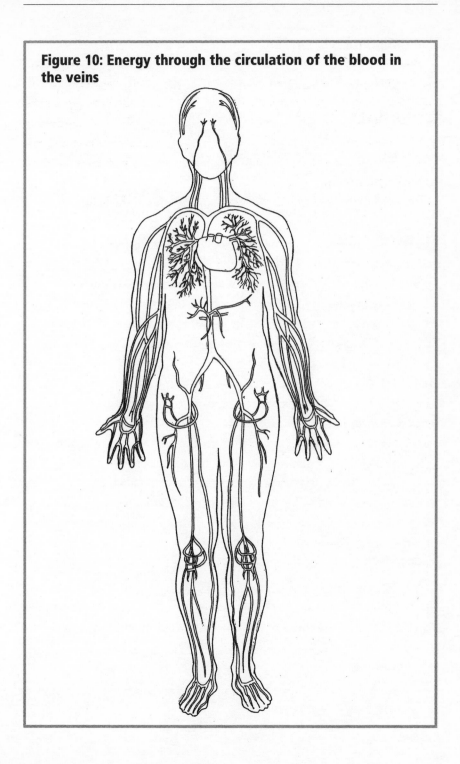

Figure 10: Energy through the circulation of the blood in the veins

The Lymphatic System

The lymph vessels provide a network of channels running alongside arteries and veins with a threefold function:

Protection: guards internal organs by producing lymphocytes and antigens to destroy harmful microrganisms.

Transport: carries oxygen and nutrients to all the cells of the body.

Drainage: returns waste fluids from all the cells of the body into the subclavian veins that arise in the heart.

The vessels carry lymph – a straw-coloured fluid containing plasma (blood fluid) and lymphocytes (white blood cells).

The lymph nodes are small knots of tissues, between 1–25mm long, which act as filters to prevent foreign particles from entering the bloodstream, and produce lymphocytes. The main sites are in the tonsils, armpits, spleen and groin. Figure 11 shows the arrangement of the major lymphatic vessels in the body.

Respiration

The respiratory process takes place when there is an exchange of gases in the lungs, in which oxygen is inhaled and carbon dioxide exhaled. This process regulates the sequence of change through the control of the breath. The exchange of gases – the uptake of oxygen and the discharge of carbon dioxide – maintains the life of the body providing it with its essential strength and ability to survive in the world. The respiratory system becomes the support for consciousness that is renewed at every breath, sustaining life until it removes itself from the physical domain.

The components of the respiratory system (see figure 12) are:

Nose and mouth: air drawn in through the nose and the mouth is moistened by blood vessels near the nasal cavity. Hairs in the nose stop foreign particles entering the lungs.

Throat (pharynx): muscular tube; passageway for air and food.

Voice box (larynx): air passage between pharynx and lungs; also produces vocal sounds.

Figure 11: Energy through the lymphatic system

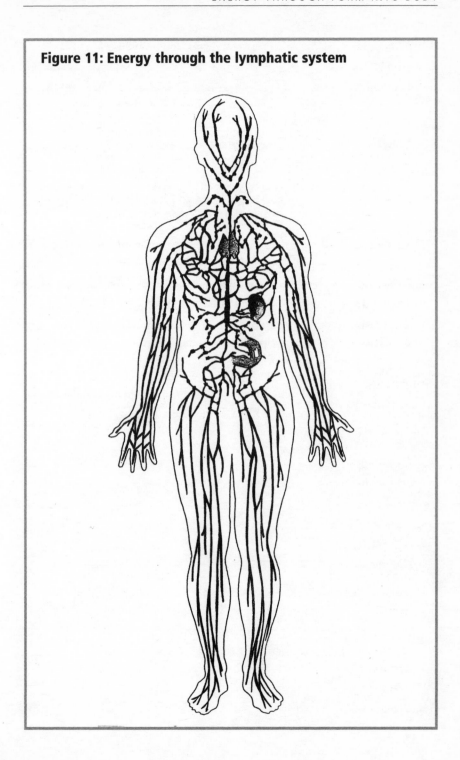

Windpipe (trachea):	air passage between larynx and bronchi.
Bronchi:	two main pathways branching off the trachea into the lungs, further dividing throughout the lungs into bronchioles.
Lungs:	spongy honeycombed organ receiving inhaled air.
Alveoli:	air sacs in the lungs where the exchange of gases takes place between oxygen and carbon dioxide. The alveoli allow the gases to pass in and out of the bloodstream as the linings are minute blood vessels.
Diaphragm:	dome-shaped muscle attached to the ribs at the sides and to the breastbone at the front of the chest.
Ribs:	curved bones providing a case around the lungs to protect them and other internal organs.
Intercostal muscles:	muscles between the ribs providing elasticity to the ribcage for inhalation and exhalation.

With inhalation the diaphragm muscle contracts and flattens to decrease pressure in the lungs and draw in air including oxygen. With exhalation the diaphragm relaxes, increasing pressure in the lungs, causing expellation of air including carbon dioxide.

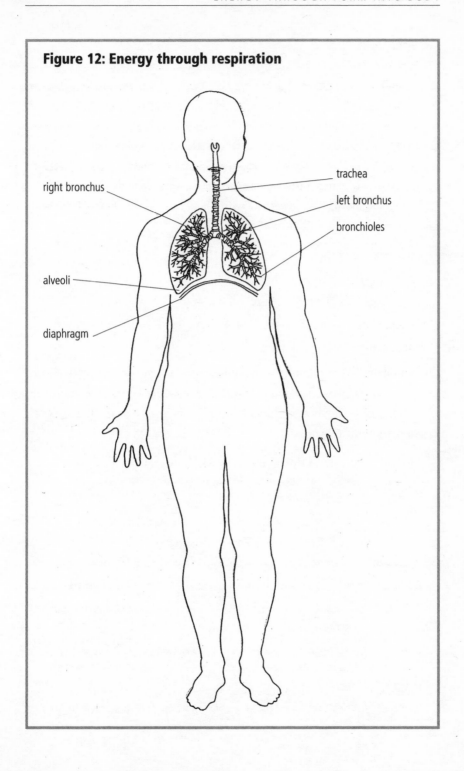

Figure 12: Energy through respiration

right bronchus

trachea

left bronchus

bronchioles

alveoli

diaphragm

Adaptation

The adaptation process operates through the endocrine system, which consists of a series of ductless glands that secrete hormones directly into the bloodstream (see figure 13). This system stimulates change. Just as there are seven layers in the aura, seven major chakras, and seven pairs of meridians, so there are seven major glands in the endocrine system that release hormones into the bloodstream. 'Hormone' means to set in motion, and the hormones that are secreted by the endocrine glands into the bloodstream enable changes to take place.

The endocrine glands co-ordinate with the nervous system to regulate a wide range of important functions including:

- ◆ formation of the physical body;
- ◆ control of the volume of body fluids;
- ◆ control of body temperature;
- ◆ stimulation of the digestive system;
- ◆ control of the reproductive system;
- ◆ protection against infection, trauma, bleeding and dehydration; and
- ◆ control of emotional and psychological attitudes.

The Endocrine Glands

Pineal: secretes the hormone melatonin which governs the brain's perception of day and night so that it can adjust biorhythms accordingly.

Pituitary: secretes hormones which affect growth, sexual development and control of other endocrine glands.

Thyroid: secretes thyroxine which regulates the rate of metabolism.

Thymus: secretes thymosin which is responsible for immunity.

Adrenal: secretes adrenaline which contributes to the fight/flight response.

Pancreas: secretes insulin which controls the body's absorption and storage of glucose.

Gonads: secretes hormones responsible for sexual development – oestrogen and progesterone in women; testosterone in men.

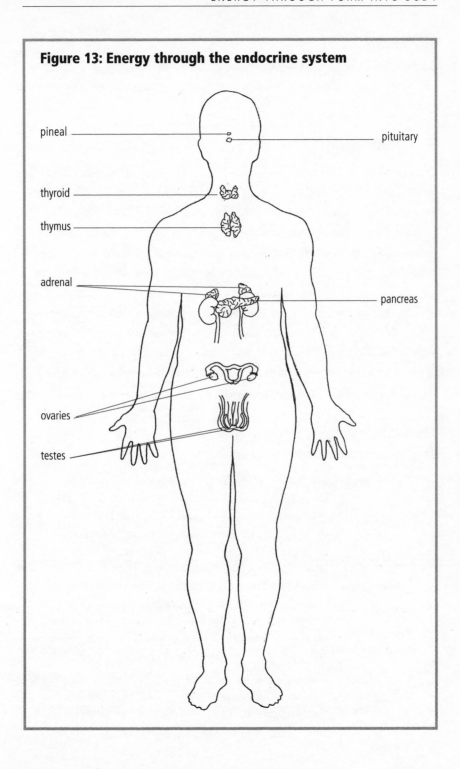

Figure 13: Energy through the endocrine system

pineal — pituitary

thyroid

thymus

adrenal — pancreas

ovaries

testes

Sensation

The components in the sensation process consist of:

- the brain;
- the central nervous system;
- the autonomic nervous system.

The brain acts as the headquarters where all nerve reactions are processed. This process senses the need for change either consciously through the central nervous system which operates along the head and spine, or automatically through the autonomic nervous system which operates along the hypothalamus, below which the pituitary gland, the master gland of the endocrine system, is located. In this way the mind and body are receptive to the sensations they experience from both the internal and external environments.

The nervous system becomes the transmitter for consciousness, the means by which the impulses sensed are converted into responsive action. The five senses of hearing, sight, smell, taste and touch operate through the five faculties of consciousness instinct, feeling, intellect, imagination and intuition to make the system fully alert (see figures 14 and 15).

The Brain

The brain consists of the following structures:

Cerebrum: also known as the forebrain, the seat of intelligence, the cerebrum controls voluntary movement, and receives and interprets conscious sensations. It is divided into two hemispheres. The left side controls the right side of the body and is associated with analytical, sequential and structured functions. The right hemisphere controls the left side of the body and is associated with initiative, creative and flexible responses. It is arranged in convoluted folds and the outer layer of grey matter contains nerve cells while the inner layer of white matter contains nerve fibres.

Cerebellum: also known as the hindbrain, the cerebellum controls muscle and sustains balance. It lies below and behind the cerebrum with an outer layer of grey matter and an inner layer of white matter.

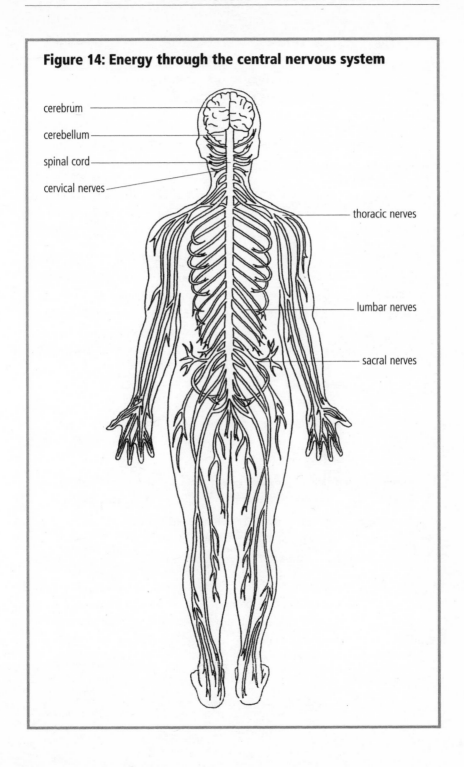

Figure 14: Energy through the central nervous system

cerebrum

cerebellum

spinal cord

cervical nerves

thoracic nerves

lumbar nerves

sacral nerves

Medulla
oblongata: also known as the midbrain, it acts as a link between
the brain and the spinal cord. It connects the brain
with the central nervous system and the autonomic
nervous system. Forms the lowest part of the brain stem

The brain is protected by the cranium (skull), three layers of membrane called
the meninges and cerebrospinal fluid – a straw-coloured fluid that flows through
the brain and the spinal cord.

The Central Nervous System

The central nervous system (see figure 14) is made up of the following structures:

Brain: the command centre for all the senses.

Nerves: bundles of nerve fibres carry messages to and from the
brain: sensory nerves carry messages from the body to
the brain; motor nerves carry messages from the brain
to the body; peripheral nerves carry messages from the
brain and the vertebrae of the spinal cord into the
body systems exerting conscious control over muscles
and subconscious, involuntary control over the body
organs.

Spinal cord: provides reflexes in response to internal and external
charges and transmits nerve messages through the
cerebrospinal fluid.

Cerebrospinal   acts as a shock absorber and circulates nutrients
fluid: filtered from the blood.

Vertebrae: bones of the spine which protect the spinal cord.
There are 33 pairs of vertebrae:

cervical – 7
thoracic – 12
lumbar – 5
sacrum – 5
coccyx – 4 (2 fused)

The Autonomic Nervous System

This part of the nervous system is responsible for controlling the activities of the body that are outside our conscious control such as heartbeat, digestion, the iris of the eye, expansion and contraction of small blood vessels, and sweat-gland secretions. It consists of the sympathetic and parasympathetic nerves. The sympathetic and the parasympathetic systems complement one another, although they may appear to be in opposition in their effects. The sympathetic works when an immediate response is required, such as in the 'fight or flight' reaction, whilst the parasympathetic operates to stabilize the system, as in the response 'rest and repose', for example in times of sleep, rest or digestion.

Sympathetic: stimulate organs;

contract muscles;

produce adrenaline and noradrenaline.

Parasympathetic: settle the organs;

relax muscles;

produce acetylcholine, the neurotransmitter that activates nerve cells.

Figure 15 shows which parts of the autonomic system control different bodily functions.

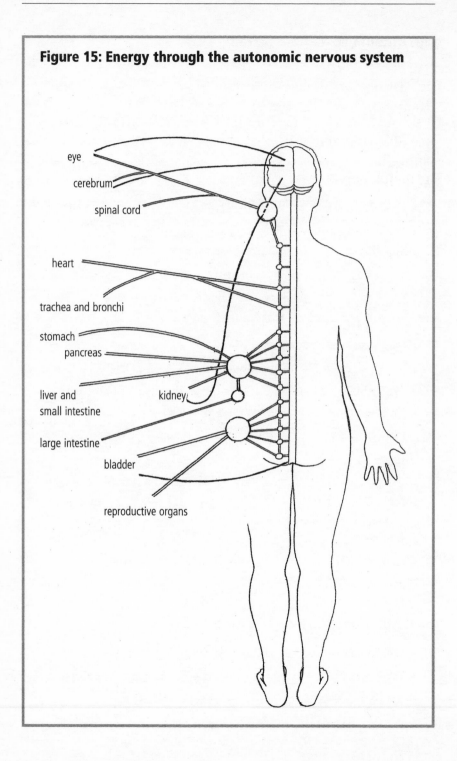

Figure 15: Energy through the autonomic nervous system

eye

cerebrum

spinal cord

heart

trachea and bronchi

stomach

pancreas

liver and
small intestine

kidney

large intestine

bladder

reproductive organs

Working with your Body Systems

The Articulation Process – Moving

- Why is it beneficial to take some form of exercise every day?
- What are the benefits to you (a) physically (b) mentally?

The Regulation Process – Flowing

- Observe your body fluids (a) urine (b) sweat (c) menstrual blood.
- What do they tell you about your state of health?
- How can you tell if you are dehydrated?
- What is the treatment for dehydration?

The Digestive Process – Absorbing

- How important is food to you?
- Is eating (a) a function (b) an indulgence (c) a problem (d) a celebration
- Do you enjoy planning, cooking and sharing food?
- Do you sit down to eat regular meals?

The Circulatory Process – Pulsating

- Use a stethoscope to listen to the sound of your heart beating. Place two fingers at the top of the wrist, or the side of the larynx to feel your pulse.
- Examine your tongue – find out its connection to your heart.
- Do you love your heart?

The Respiratory Process – Inspiring

- Feel your breath on the back of your hand.
- Take three breaths in (a) the throat (b) the chest (c) the abdomen.
- Which breath best supports (a) speaking loudly (b) singing?
- What is the most comfortable body position for breathing?

The Adaptation Process – Changing

- How swift are your responses?

- How efficient is your immune system?

- How adaptable are you to changes in circumstances?

- How often do you feel tired during your day?

The Sensation Process – Responding

- Examine your senses: (a) hearing (b) sight (c) smell (d) taste (e) touch.

- Which are (a) the strongest (b) the weakest?

- How can you develop each sense?

The Tao

Tao produced the one

The one produced the two

The two produced the three

And the three produced the ten thousand things

And ten thousand things carry the Yin

And embrace the Yang

And through the blending of the Qi

They achieve harmony.

LAO TSU

1.4

Energy through the Seven Pairs of Meridians

Energy is channelled into the body processes through the 14 meridians, 12 of which flow on each side of the body, whilst the remaining 2 traverse its centre. The meridians act as pathways for the vital force, or *chi*, and connect to specific structures and functions of the organs in the body. They can be accessed through such practices as acupuncture, reflexology and shiatsu, and cultivated through such exercises as chi gung, aikido and t'ai chi.

Meridians contain the free-flowing energy (*chi*) that is both subtle and yet substantial. This can be observed by modern technological methods, such as Kirlian photography or bioelectrical machines that measure skin resistance. The meridians contain specific contact points through which energy can be influenced in order to move, stimulate or sedate both the physical organs and the energy itself.

All the meridians come from one continuous source, dividing into the 14 channels that work in pairs. In each pair, one is classified as yin and the other as yang, according to the nature and function of the organs to which they connect. Energy in the meridians may be felt at the pulse in the wrists, where different positions relate to each organ and meridian – it is said that it takes at least 20 years to become sensitized to all the subtleties in the points of the pulse.

With each meridian there is a two-hour period during which energy is at its fullest and equally, twelve hours later there is a corresponding two-hour period when it is at its lowest. The flow of energy through the meridians is cyclical,

Energy through the seven pairs of meridians

Meridian	Element	Source	Time	Function	Emotion	Sound
Lung	Metal-	Yin	3am–5am	Respiration	Grief	Sss
Large intestine		Yang	5am–7am	Elimination	Acceptance	Weeping
Stomach	Earth	Yang	7am–9am	Digestion	Anxiety	Hoo
Spleen		Yin	9am–11am	Transformation	Sympathy	Singing
Heart	Fire	Yin	11am–1pm	Circulation	Hate	Her
Small intestine		Yang	1pm–3pm	Absorption	Joy	Laughing
Bladder	Water	Yang	3pm–5pm	Urination	Fear	Chway
Kidneys		Yin	5pm–7pm	Regulation	Calmness	Groaning
Heart protector	Fire	Yin	7pm–9pm	Protection	Threat	Her
Triple heater		Yang	9pm–11pm	Heat control	Safety	Laughing
Gall bladder	Wood	Yang	11pm–1am	Purification	Anger	Hsu
Liver		Yin	1am–3am	Metabolism	Generosity	Shouting
Conception vessel	–	Yin		Controls all yin meridians	Receptive	–
			All the time			
Governor vessel	–	Yang		Controls all yang meridians	Active	–

moving clockwise throughout the 24-hour period, and this can be seen in the illustration of the 24-hour cycle of energy through the meridians. When energy is at its peak, then symptoms relating to excess energy can become most apparent. Symptoms relating to deficiency show themselves when energy is at its lowest ebb (see figure 16).

Figure 16: The 24-hour cycle of energy through the meridians

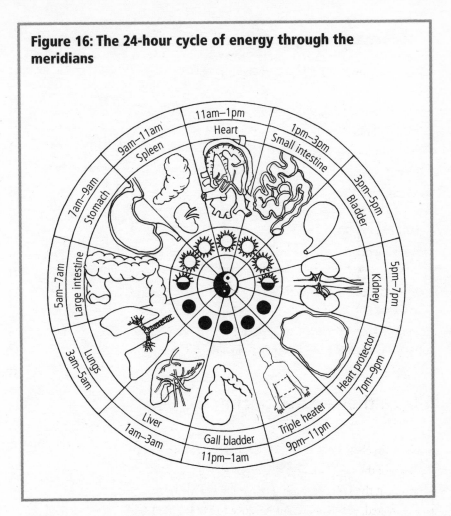

The meridians can be sensed either in the hands or in the feet, with each digit relating to a specific meridian. In this way the energy state of the individual organs can be ascertained. The meridians are ruled by the emperor, the energy of the heart, and shielded by the emperor's bodyguard, the energy of the pericardium, which protects the heart. Led by the prime minister, the energy of the lungs, all the other meridians, which are called the ministers, serve specific organs of the body. The meridians are supported by the two civil servants, known as the governor and conception vessels, which direct energy down the back and up the front of the spine to uphold constitution (see figure 17).

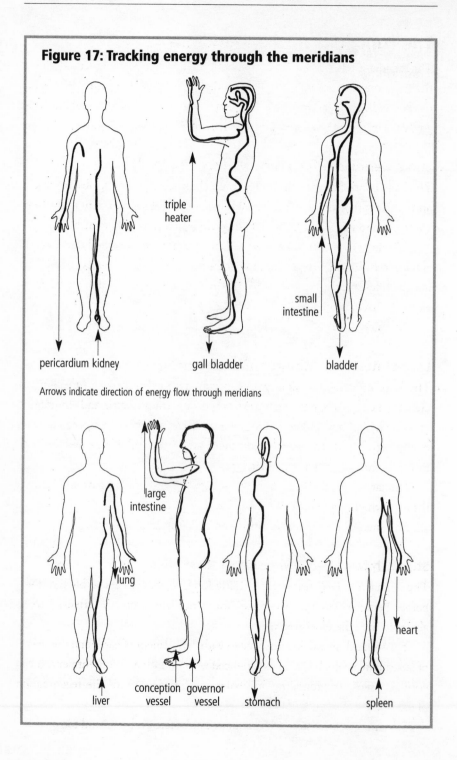

Figure 17: Tracking energy through the meridians

triple
heater

small
intestine

pericardium kidney   gall bladder   bladder

Arrows indicate direction of energy flow through meridians

large
intestine

lung

heart

liver   conception governor   stomach   spleen
               vessel   vessel

The Functions of the Meridians

The meridians reflect the functions of both the body and the mind, according to the traditions that originated in India and were developed in China. According to the traditional laws of Five Element Acupuncture all the meridians are governed by one of five elements which are: metal, earth, fire, water and wood.

Lung Meridian – The Prime Minister

The lungs control the breath through their ability to inhale air to absorb oxygen, and exhale carbon dioxide. They enable oxygenated blood to be sent to the heart via the pulmonary vein, so that it can be circulated throughout the body.

The lung meridian is associated with the element of metal and the season of autumn, which can be experienced with a sense of drawing in and even loss. This may manifest psychologically through the lung meridian as grief; physically it expresses itself as the uptake of oxygen.

The energy of the lung meridian can be felt in the thumb.

Large Intestine – Minister of Transport

The large intestine meridian works in conjunction with that of the lung. It creates an empty space through the transporting, transforming and eliminating of both physical and psychological waste products, so that the lungs can draw in new energy. The diaphragm controls the actions of both the lungs and the large intestine through its muscular activity.

The large intestine meridian is associated with containment and release, through which grief may be processed and eliminated.

The energy of the large intestine can be felt in the forefinger.

Stomach Meridian – Minister of the Mill

The stomach is responsible for holding food, so that it can be broken down before being passed into the small intestine, where micronutrients can be absorbed into the bloodstream.

The stomach meridian is associated with the element of earth and the season of late summer, which can be experienced with warmth and contentment. It can convey a sense of grounding and balance, so necessary for the regeneration of energy.

The energy of the stomach meridian can be felt in the second toe.

Spleen Meridian – Minister of the Granary

The spleen meridian works in close conjunction with that of the stomach. Whilst the stomach takes food downwards, the spleen releases the energy from it upwards, in the form of blood which sustains life.

When there is an excess of energy in the spleen it may result in a person being 'splenetic' or hot-blooded, leading to impulsive and ungrounded responses.

The energy of the spleen meridian can be felt at the back of the big toe.

Heart Meridian – Emperor of all the Organs

The heart controls the circulation and distribution of the blood. It can be likened to the throne of the kingdom, through which all the commands for sustaining life are directed. The heart requires pure energy in order to fulfil its function most effectively.

The heart is associated with the element of fire and the season of summer, which can be experienced with expansiveness and enthusiasm.

The energy of the heart meridian can be felt in the little finger.

Small Intestine – Minister of Reception

The small intestine meridian works in conjunction with that of the heart. Its primary function is to separate the pure from the impure, so that physically the food required by the body is utilized, and what is not needed is eliminated through the bowels.

This process of discernment is also reflected in the functions of the mind, especially within an emotional context. When there is a conflict of unexpressed or unresolved feelings it can lead to either an inflated or deflated attitude to life which prevents choices from being made within a realistic context.

The energy of the small intestine meridian can be felt on the tip of the little finger.

Bladder Meridian – Minister of the Reservoir

This is the largest meridian in the body. Its function is to control the distribution of water, the primary constituent of life. Water moves through the body in waves, like the tides of the ocean, and the bladder meridian is required to control its power.

The bladder meridian is associated with the element of water and the season of winter, with its sense of restriction and isolation, which can be experienced by feeling alone and adrift.

The energy of the bladder meridian can be felt on the outer part of the little toe.

Kidney Meridian – Minister of Power

The kidney meridian works in conjunction with that of the bladder. Its primary function is to release the vital force that sustains the body, mind and soul in the physical form. This relates physically to the function of adrenaline which is produced by the adrenal glands. The ovaries and testes, which are concerned with the reproduction of life, are known as the external kidneys. The physical function of the kidneys is to maintain the balance of water and mineral salts in the body.

Imbalance in the kidney meridian can be associated with fear, which may reveal itself in excessive urination.

The energy of the kidney meridian can be felt on the inner part of the little toe.

Heart Protector Meridian – The Emperor's Bodyguard

The heart protector meridian relates physiologically to the pericardium, which is the membranous sac that envelopes the heart, to guard it from harm.

The heart protector meridian, together with the heart, is associated with the element of fire and the season of summer. Physically it acts as a filter between all the organs and the heart, in order to preserve its essential function. Psychologically it relates to the experience of love, and in particular to sexual intimacy, as opposed to the raw reproductive urge that is generated through the kidney meridian.

The energy of the heart protector meridian can be felt in the middle finger.

Triple Heater Meridian – Minister of Dykes and Dredges

The triple heater meridian works in conjunction with the heart protector, to control the body temperature in the three cavities of the torso: the thorax, the abdomen, and the pelvis. It is linked with the hypothalamus, which acts as the bridge between the nervous system and the endocrine glands and which controls the series of chemical changes through which the system maintains itself.

The triple heater is associated with warmth in all areas of life, in the body, mind and soul.

The energy of the triple heater meridian can be felt on the ring finger.

Gall bladder Meridian – Honourable Minister

The gall bladder stores and secretes bile for the breakdown of fats, which in their purest form are formidable sources of energy. Unlike other systems the gall bladder works only with the pure material produced by the lymphatic system, which clears the toxic by-products of metabolism.

A build-up of impure material, either physically or psychologically, can lead to feelings of frustration and resentment. This can lead to an inability to make decisions because there is not enough access to the pure energy required to formulate and implement plans, both of which are key functions of the gall bladder meridian.

The gall bladder meridian is associated with the element of wood and the season of spring, with its abundance of renewed energy and life.

The energy of the gall bladder meridian can be felt on the fourth toe.

The Liver Meridian – Chief of Staff

The liver acts as the 'butler' to the brain, directing the flow of energy throughout the body. It filters, detoxifies, nourishes, replenishes and stores blood. It also controls the peripheral nervous system, which regulates the movements of the muscles, ligaments and tendons, enabling the nerve messages from the brain to be carried to their destinations.

When the energy of the liver meridian is thwarted physically or psychologically in its function it becomes associated with anger, which is magnified by the increased energy of spring. It has a powerful role to play in the generation of energy, and needs to be well cared for in order to be able to carry out its work effectively.

The energy of the liver meridian can be felt in the big toe.

Conception Vessel – The Female Civil Servant

The conception vessel governs the activity in all the yin organs, which are the lungs, spleen, heart, kidneys, heart protector and liver. The yin meridians are seen as negative, passive, female, interior and dark. The conception vessel relates to the flow of emotions, and to creativity in all its aspects. Running up the front of the spine, from the pelvic cavity to the lower jaw, there is a connecting point at the base of the sternum which affects all the yin meridians.

Governor Vessel – The Male Civil Servant

The governor vessel governs the activity of all the yang organs, which are the large intestine, stomach, small intestine, bladder, triple heater and gall bladder, which are seen as positive, active, male, exterior and light. The governor vessel relates to the strength of the will and the ability to sustain it. Running up the back of the spine, from the pelvic cavity over the head and ending below the nose, there is a connecting point on the top of the head which affects all the yang meridians.

The Meridians and Related Health Problems

Each meridian follows an appointed track along the physical body, and seemingly disconnected symptoms of illness may find their connection through these pathways. As the meridians work in pairs there may be a crossover of symptoms in each pair of meridians, so that an imbalance of energy in a yang meridian will affect its yin partner, and vice versa. Observing the flow of the meridians through the body clarifies the relationship between the structures and functions of the body systems, as well as deepening the understanding of their relationships with one another. For example, this link may be seen in relation to the liver meridian, which begins in the big toe, where gout often occurs when the liver has been overwhelmed by an excess of fatty foods and alcohol. Similarly it may be seen in relation to the heart, where the lack of oxygen causes pain to spread through the chest, across the shoulder, under and down the arm, and into the fingers of the hand, following the track of the heart meridian pathway. It is always helpful to consider the location then of the meridians with regards to illness, in particular to aid the discovery of the underlying cause.

The meridians and related health problems

Meridian	Appointment	Pole	Begins	Ends	Disorders
Lung	Prime Minister	Yin	Clavicle	Thumb	Shoulder pain Stiff forearms Skin problems Wrist disorders Warts Moles Thumbnail problems
Large intestine	Minister of Transport	Yang	Forefinger	By the nose	Forefinger pain Wrist problems Tennis elbow Shoulder pain Throat problems Cold sores Nose problems
Stomach	Minister of the Mill	Yang	Under the eye	Second toe	Eye problems Teeth problems Lung problems Digestive problems Menstrual problems Knee problems Second-toe pain
Spleen	Minister of the Granary	Yin	Big toe	Under the armpit	Bunions Phlebitis Psoriasis Menstrual problems Digestive problems Breast problems Underarm problems
Heart	Emperor of all the Organs	Yin	Armpit	Little finger	Pain in armpit Inner-arm pain/weakness Palpitations Angina Chest pains Throat disorders Little-finger pain
Small intestine	Minister of Reception	Yang	Little finger	Outer corner of eye	Little-finger pains Swollen glands in neck Trigeminal neuralgia Tinnitus/deafness Heart problems Digestive problems Trigeminal neuralgia
Bladder	Minister of the Reservoir	Yang	Inner corner of eye	Little toe	Headaches Sinus problems Hair loss Back problems Haemorrhoids Varicose veins Athlete's foot

The meridians and related health problems [cont]

Meridian	Appointment	Pole	Begins	Ends	Disorders
Kidney	Minister of Power	Yin	Sole of the foot	Breastbone	Foot problems Inner-ankle problems Sexual problems Bladder problems Hip problems Digestive problems Chest problems
Heart protector	Emperor's Bodyguard	Yin	Chest	Second finger	Heart problems Endocrine problems Swollen armpits Eczema Arthritis Carpal tunnel syndrome Second-finger pain
Triple heater	Minister of Dykes and Dredges	Yang	Third finger	Head	Third-finger problems Eczema Arthritis Ear problems Eye pain Headaches Thoracic/upper abdominal/ lower abdominal problems
Gall bladder	Honourable Minister	Yang	Outer corner of the eye	Fourth toe	Migraines Shoulder pains Asthma Shingles Hip problems Knee problems Fourth-toe pains
Liver	Chief of Staff	Yin	Big toe	Under the nipple	Big-toe problems e.g. gout Varicose veins Genital problems Liver problems Digestive problems Eye problems Chest tightness
Conception vessel	Female Civil Servant	Yin	Pelvic cavity	Lower jaw	Back problems – in the front of the spine relating to 'won't' power Fear of communication, commitment, choice, change, confrontation, freedom, family
Governor vessel	Male Civil Servant	Yang	Pelvic cavity	Upper lip	Back problems – in the back of the spine relating to 'will' power 'backbone', 'back off' 'back against', 'back log', 'background', 'backward', 'back-facing'

59

Reflection on the seven pairs of meridians

- Sit quietly and take one or two breaths.
- Ask to be opened up to your inner sight and inner voice.
- Ask for permission to enter each meridian.
- Allow the process to unfold as it wills.
- Chant the sounds into each pair of meridians.
- Breathe silence into the two vessels.
- Give thanks for your experience.
- Take one or two deep breaths.
- Check that you feel grounded.
- Record any impressions from your reflections.

Name	Sound	Transliteration
Lung	Sss	Fei
Large intestine		Da chang
Stomach	Hoo	Wei
Spleen		Pi
Heart	Her	Xin
Small intestine		Xiao chang
Bladder	Chway	Pang guang
Kidneys		Schen
Heart protector	Her	Xin bao
Triple heater		San jiao
Gall bladder	Hsu	Dan
Liver		Gan
Governor vessel		Du mo
Conception vessel		Ren mo

1.5

Energy through the Seven Chakras

You walk, as it were, round yourself
in the revelation.

XENOS CLARKE

The meridians receive energy from the chakras. Just as there are seven colours in the rainbow which reflect the seven bodies of energy in all living beings, so there are seven chakras which revolve at varying speeds along the length of the human body. These vortices of energy reflect the seven levels of the auric body: physical, etheric, astral, mind, soul, spirit and divine.

Each chakra is connected to a major nerve plexus and glandular centre within the endocrine system. Overactivity in a particular chakra can lead to inflammatory disease and underactivity can cause degenerative illness in the part of the body from which its energy derives.

The understanding of the interaction of the chakras, the nerves and the glands is profoundly complex and is still being researched. This can be developed by applying modern scientific methods to explore the links between the ancient tradition of chakras and the anatomy and physiology of the nervous and endocrine systems. Such investigation can reveal what relevance they have to one another, both physically and psychologically, in the understanding of health and the maintenance of well-being. The following table summarizes how each chakra affects the physical and mental processes.

Energy through the seven chakras

Chakra	Location	Colour	Gland	Body action	Mind function	Sound
Crown	Top of the head	Purple	Pineal	Sensation	Self-consciousness	
Brow	Between the eyes	Blue	Pituitary	Adaptation	Self-responsibility	Om
Throat	Neck	Turquoise	Thyroid	Respiration	Self-expression	Ham
Heart	Chest	Green	Thymus	Circulation	Self-acceptance	Yam
Solar plexus	Diaphragm	Yellow	Pancreas	Digestion	Self-worth	Ram
Sacral	Below umbilicus	Orange	Gonads	Regulation	Self-respect	Vam
Base	Base of spine	Red	Adrenals	Articulation	Self-awareness	Lam

The Seven Chakras

1 The Crown Chakra – I am Conscious of Myself

The crown chakra is located on the top of the head, and usually presents itself first in the birth of a child in the 'crowning' during the second stage of labour. It reverberates to the colour purple, radiating richness, absorption and majestic strength. This chakra relates to the uppermost levels of consciousness, where insights may be given beyond the normal conditions of relativity. It is here that heightened states of awareness may appear, such as mystical and psychic experiences.

This chakra is linked to the pineal gland, a small cone-like structure situated in the mid-brain, which secretes serotonin, a hormone which has a profound influence on our feelings.

The essential purpose of the crown chakra is the development of self-consciousness, which arises through the relationship between the senses of the body and the faculties of the mind. The crown chakra opens up to energy from many sources without limitation. It is usually lightly closed so that it can filter the flow of energy into the brow chakra where the mind undertakes its interpretive functions in the processes of the brain. Through the experience and exploration of consciousness comes a sense of self, which directs and informs us in all our thoughts and actions.

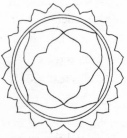

Figure 18: Sahasrara – crown chakra

2 The Brow Chakra – I Reflect

The brow chakra is located between the eyes, and is referred to as the third eye. It reverberates to the colour blue, radiating profound tranquillity, and relates to all the faculties of consciousness as they make themselves known through the insights of the mind.

Figure 19: Ajna – brow chakra

This chakra is linked to the pituitary gland, which acts as the conductor and controller to all the other glands in the endocrine system. It is the size of a pea, and located behind the bridge of the nose.

The essential purpose of the brow chakra is the development of self-reflection which encourages a willingness to accept that we, and not others, are ultimately accountable for our lives and what happens in them.

3 The Throat Chakra – I Express

The throat chakra is located in the centre of the neck and reverberates to the colour turquoise, radiating fluency and illumination. It relates to the need for communication, to clarify and articulate instinctive, emotional, analytical, imaginative and intuitive thought.

This chakra is linked to the thyroid and parathyroid glands, found on either side of the trachea, which control the metabolic rate, the continuous series of chemical changes through which life is sustained in the living body.

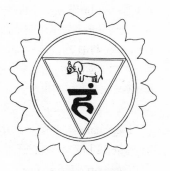

Figure 20: Visuddha – throat chakra

The essential purpose of the throat chakra is the development of self-expression, which is the outer face of mindfulness. The inner face is the willingness to observe the thoughts as they arise, letting go of what is reactionary and negative, vocalizing what is clear and truthful if expression is required.

4 The Heart Chakra – I Accept

The heart chakra is located in both the centre of the chest and the energy system. When the energy flows unimpeded there is a balance between the upper

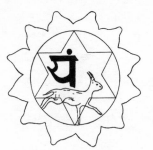

Figure 21: Anahata –
heart chakra

and the lower chakras, utilizing head, heart and body in response to the needs of the moment. Excessive energy in the upper chakras results in thought processes that cannot be transformed into effective action, causing the experience of being 'high' or of not being grounded. In the lower chakras, a surplus of energy results in impulsive and provocative action which may be described as a 'mindless' response. The heart chakra acts as a gateway between the two, allowing a flow of energy which is necessary to maintain balance and harmony throughout the healthy system. This chakra reverberates to the colour green, radiating strength and renewal. It relates to the experience of love, which can be seen as the opening of the heart, and is at the centre of a meaningful life.

The heart chakra relates both to the circulatory and immune systems. It is linked to the thymus gland, which lies behind the breastbone, activating and controlling the immune system whose work is to protect the organism from harm.

The essential purpose of the heart chakra is the development of self-acceptance. This allows an opening up to the movement of unconditional love, which requires neither proof nor power to make itself known, but only a means to express itself. The more deeply this love is experienced, the more powerfully the heart chakra turns, drawing in energy from all the other chakras. Such love is not fixed by conditions but moves in response to the opening of the heart as a result of experiencing love.

5 The Solar Plexus Chakra – I Absorb

The solar plexus chakra is located in the diaphragm, the sheet of smooth muscle which divides the thorax from the abdomen, and reverberates to the colour yellow, radiating brightness and freshness. It relates to the absorption and assimilation of food in the digestive system as well as the absorption of experiences and the emotional reactions to them.

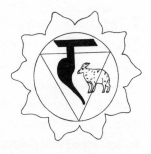

Figure 22: Manipuraka –
solar plexus chakra

It is linked with the pancreas, the tongue-shaped gland that lies below and behind the stomach, which produces insulin to convert carbohydrates into glucose.

The essential purpose of this chakra is the development of a self-worth which values the gift of life and is nourished by it. The gift of life itself is priceless, but using it effectively requires an appreciation of its value, so that its full worth is not squandered.

6 The Sacral Chakra – I Create

The sacral chakra is located below the umbilical cord and reverberates to the colour orange, radiating creativity and artistry. The sacral chakra relates to relationships of every form, from the pairing of couples to the connection between the creator and the creative endeavour of any type, whether artistic, scientific or practical in nature.

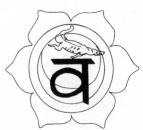

Figure 23: Svadisthana – sacral chakra

This chakra is linked both to the adrenal glands which produce adrenalin to stimulate the urinary system and to the gonads which activate the reproductive system, producing a predominance of oestrogen and progesterone in the female and testosterone in the male. Its essential purpose is self-respect, which comes from the ability to acknowledge the perspective of others as well as our own, giving both their due accord so that we are not fixed or limited by either, but able to adapt to changing circumstances with a commitment to create the best conditions for ourselves.

7 The Base/Root Chakra – I Stand

The base chakra is located, as its name suggests, at the base of the spine and reverberates to the colour red, radiating energy, fire and depth. It relates to the need to be grounded, to feel rooted in the earth and established in the world, and to be connected with the present moment through the harmony of mind and body.

It is linked with the adrenal glands which

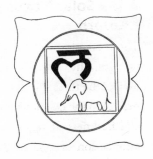

Figure 24: Muladhara – base chakra

function according to the physical and psychological needs of the person. If they become overstimulated, through, for example, an habitual state of constriction, they cease to generate sufficient energy for general health and well-being. This may reveal itself in restlessness, exhaustion, lack of libido, infertility, and frequent accidents or illness.

The essential purpose of this chakra is the development of a self-awareness throughout the physical body which results from its alignment with the mind, so that both are fully attuned to one another. In this way, a person stands in the centre of their own field of energy, able to access all its resources, acknowledging its interconnection with all other forms of energy and yet uniquely accountable for personal life experience.

Within the context of spiritual healing it is vital when working with the chakras to start from the crown and work downwards to the base. If work begins at the base it can draw toxic energies which may have accumulated there into the whole system, causing profound problems in the physical, psychological and spiritual levels of consciousness.

Reflection on the Seven Chakras

- ◆ Sit quietly.
- ◆ Take one or two deep breaths.
- ◆ Ask to be opened up to your inner sight and inner voice.
- ◆ Ask for permission to enter each chakra.
- ◆ Allow the process to unfold as it wills.
- ◆ Breathe the following colours into each chakra (see page 67).
- ◆ Give thanks for your experience.
- ◆ Take one or two deep breaths.
- ◆ Check that you feel grounded.
- ◆ Record any impressions from your reflections.

Chant the sound of the chakra through each colour

Sound	Colour	Chakra	
—	Purple into the crown	Sahasrara – crown	
Om	Blue into the brow	Ajna – brow	
Ham	Turquoise into the throat	Visuddha – throat	
Yam	Green into the heart	Anahata – heart	
Ram	Yellow into the solar plexus	Manipuraka – solar plexus	
Vam	Orange into the sacral	Svadisthana – sacral	
Lam	Red into the base	Muladhara – base	

1.6

Energy through the Seven Bodies of the Aura

Light reveals colour: colour reveals Light.

ANON

The seven bodies of energy that surround every organism and make up its electromagnetic field are often referred to as the aura. The word aura comes from the Greek '*avra*' meaning 'breeze', and can be seen through clairvoyant vision as shimmering in the air. The aura of the human being is egg-shaped. It extends several feet around the human form, but shrinks when there is physical or psychological imbalance.

Currents of energy circulate through it: the horizontal currents absorb and carry the life forces from the atmosphere and dispose of etheric waste products, and the vertical ones relate to the autonomic nervous system. Each level of energy is either seen or visualized through a colour, beginning with the red of the physical body and ending with purple which is associated with the divine.

The colours and characteristics of the aura reflect those of the chakras, revealing the characteristics of the energy which circulates through them.

Purple is associated with royalty, and this can be seen in the regalia of the monarch and the vestments of the Church. As in a rainbow, purple fades into white, and this is represented in nature in the petals of certain flowers like pansies. Its presence is both subtle and stilling.

Blue is associated with scholarship and authority, as in the classic school dress and the uniform of the police. In nature it can be found in the skies just before dark. Its presence is calming and peaceful.

Turquoise is associated with the voice in all its forms of expression, as in the use of lapis lazuli to aid communication. In nature it can be seen in the unpolluted sea, where the water meets the land. Its presence is vibrant and expressive.

Green is associated with birth and revival, as in the tradition of the Green Man. It is represented by the lushness of natural surroundings. Its presence is expansive and harmonious.

Yellow is associated with the eating process, as in the use of yellow dock for digestive problems. In nature it can be seen in the sun that generates the heat necessary for life. Its presence is stimulating and refreshing.

Orange is associated with protection and security, as in the hazard lights of a car. In nature it can be found in the setting of the sun at the end of the day. Its presence is warming and vital.

Red is associated with love and passion as in the rose, the traditional flower of lovers. In nature it can be found in the blood that carries the life force through the body. Its presence is glowing and strengthening.

The seven bodies of energy vibrate at different rates, with the slowest vibrations occurring in the physical body, and increasing in speed as they reach into the outer energy space. These energy fields will vary in strength according to the physical and psychological state of health of each individual and the willingness to go beyond outer form into inner meaning.

The outer bodies may be seen through the visible eye, but the innermost ones can be seen only through the inner eye in a state of deep reflection or meditation. Each body has a specific function:

The Physical Body – that which appears

The physical body contains energy at a molecular level, which promotes birth, growth, decay, and renewal. The process of homeostasis, which stabilizes the structures and functions of the organism, provides the anchor for the connection of all the subsequent bodies of energy.

The Etheric Body – that which links

The etheric body contains energy at a submolecular level, which supports the exterior structure and function of the organism. It can be seen as a template of the outer form and its inner structure, linking the physical body to the incoming energies of the astral, mind, soul, spirit, and divine.

The Astral Body – that which feels

The astral body represents the emotions, which set feelings in motion. This allows the underlying information from the deeper levels of consciousness to make itself known through the other faculties of the mind.

The Mind Body – that which correlates

The mind body represents the potential for the enlightenment of consciousness in all its expressions, through the faculties of instinct, feeling, intellect, imagination and intuition. Its primary connection is with the heart, the centre through which all meaning finds its fullest expression as indicated in the saying 'going to the heart of the matter'.

The Soul Body – that which nurtures

The soul represents the receptive level of consciousness, the conjunction of spirit with matter. Spirit animates the life force and matter grounds it. Acting as a meeting place for the transcendent and the immanent energies, the soul nurtures this union.

The Spirit – that which inspires

The spirit represents the life force. It does not change of itself, because it is infinite and indestructible, but it inspires changes to take place in the subsequent bodies of energy, which are finite and flexible in their constitutions.

The Divine – that which unites

The divine is both the innermost and the outermost energy, for it effuses all that is. As that which can be named, it is the exterior face of being which is made manifest throughout all creation. Its inner face is non-manifest and beyond all human comprehension.

*   *   *

The aura is a reflection of the whole energy field, unique in composition in every being, ever changing as it reveals what is happening in the chakras, the meridians and in every cell of the body. As the aura extends above, around and below the physical form it makes contact with the energy of people, objects and places with which it comes into contact physically, psychologically and spiritually. This nexus draws everything into the web that is woven by the force of life, to hold all in being.

Reflection on the Aura

◆ Sit quietly.

◆ Take one or two breaths.

◆ Ask to be opened up to your inner sight and inner voice.

◆ Ask for permission to witness the colours of the aura.

◆ Allow the process to unfold as it wills.

◆ Absorb the colours through each body of energy.

◆ Focus on each colour through the seven levels of energy.

◆ Give thanks for your experience.

◆ Take one or two deep breaths.

◆ Check that you feel grounded.

◆ Record any impressions from your reflections.

Body	Colour
Divine	Purple
Spirit	Blue
Soul	Turquoise
Mind	Green
Astral	Yellow
Etheric	Orange
Physical	Red

1.7

Energy for the Whole Person

In being there is energy and in this energy there are forms. The more the forms of energy are explored and their mysteries unravelled, the deeper the connections that can be made between energy in its most subtle and its most manifest expressions. The ancient wisdoms of the meridians, the chakras and the auric bodies can bring a depth of understanding to the complexities of the physical functions, linking symptoms of disease to their underlying causes in the energy field.

Within this paradigm the body is no longer seen as a machine containing a series of components that operate separately from one another, but as an external manifestation of its internal activities, through all the levels of its consciousness. When the body is accepted as a mirror of the energy contained within, the whole being comes into view. When illness occurs, it is no longer seen as an isolated, disconnected experience, something to be suppressed, but as a call for help, so that the relevant adjustments to restore all the systems into a harmonious whole can be set in motion. Within this context wellness is no longer taken for granted or ignored until illness presents itself, but becomes a dynamic process in which each participant is invited to take part. It places each person in the centre of their own life, so that they can respond to their unique set of continually unfolding circumstances, with all the levels of energy that are at their disposal.

Section 2

HEALTH

2.1

Correlating Energy with Health

Energy is infinite and indestructible; health is finite and perishable. Where then is the mutual relationship between these two seemingly opposing states of being? Energy serves life at every level, from its highest expression as consciousness to its lowest presence in the anatomy and physiology of the physical form. Health in turn, serves energy, reflecting its movement or lack of it, through the seven levels which constitute the life form. Since all life forms are infused with energy they have the potential to relate both to the infinite nature of spirit through attunement, and to the finite structures of the physical world through inhabitation.

Health acts a bridge between the infinite and the finite, through the functions of the body, the thought processes of the mind, and the self-expression of the soul. By travelling along this path, what is hidden may be revealed and the source of illness uncovered. Broadening the perspective from a purely functional view of the body to include the whole being brings a growing realization that complete health is a journey of self-discovery.

During this journey it becomes apparent that we often take health for granted and only pay attention to it when illness arises. It then becomes clear that good health is a state of being that needs to be nurtured and requires co-operation from us.

It is essentially an expression of relationship: for example, the lungs with the heart, so that air can be pumped around the body; the brain with the spine, so that the messages from the nervous systems can be distributed from head to toe; and the bones with the muscles and joints, so that the framework of the body can be set in motion. The most important of these relationships is that of the human with the divine, so that all the faces of being may be encountered. It can seem to be a paradox that there is relationship when the nature of being is singular. Yet everywhere there is apparent diversity, the movement of one into two, and the relationship between them.

Life is always present in potential, but requires relationship to bring it into being in this plane of existence. The activity of life is perpetual, but at its core is stillness. From stillness comes the inspiration of being, and through movement its detailing in action. It is the harmony that resonates from the balance of stillness and action that determines health and it is important to allow both of them their place, as the inner and outer faces of the organism. The potential for well-being is renewed at every instant, maintaining all the systems and stimulating the healing processes when required. From this perspective ill health can never be attributed to one cause, such as poor nutrition, a stressful lifestyle, or a polluted environment. They may be contributory factors but they do not reveal the whole picture, giving but a partial image of what is most evident. The entirety is seen only when the whole person is taken into account.

Energy manifests itself as health when the mind, body, and soul are in harmony with one another. Working through the consciousness of energy in the seven chakras, the adjustments required to maintain this balance can be explored in seven ways:

1 Crown Chakra
This can be explored as intelligence is brought into sensation via the cerebral hormones, which in turn set the nervous systems in motion, through the five senses of the body: sound, sight, taste, touch and smell, in co-ordination with the five faculties of the mind: instinct, feelings, intellect, imagination and intuition. The faculties of the mind are made more acute by the senses of the body so that we may learn to assess ourselves fully through the intelligence which is innate in all these processes.

2 Brow Chakra

This can be explored as it works with the pituitary gland, which controls all the other glands in the body. Stress builds up when there is a failure to adjust both physically and psychologically to changing circumstances. Resistance to these holds back the ability to act spontaneously. When stress is recognized and released it allows the hormones to carry out their appointed task, which is to adapt to ever changing situations.

3 Throat Chakra

This is where the thyroid gland controls the body's metabolic rate, by communicating at a cellular level in order to stabilize the energy which has been set in motion through the endocrine system. Communication finds its most powerful exterior expression in the human voice which carries and conveys meanings of every kind. The desire to speak, to be heard and to be listened to is fundamental to the expression of meaning which is at the heart of being human.

4 Heart Chakra

This works through the thymus gland which controls the functions of the heart and the immune system. The energy that has been received through the crown chakra, set in motion through the brow chakra and stabilized in the throat, contains the vital force which animates the life form. This vital force is carried in the blood and circulated throughout the body. It is associated with the receiving and returning of love and expresses the essential vitality of being alive.

5 Solar Plexus Chakra

This is responsible for breaking down physical nutrients through the digestive system under the influence of the pancreas, keeping what is useful and discarding what is not. This process of separation on the physical plane is reflected on the emotional level as discernment, through which similar choices are made at a psychological level. When discernment is activated it encourages one to accept full responsibility for oneself.

6 Sacral Chakra

This can be explored as it regulates the urinary and reproductive systems, under the influence of the hormones: oestrogen, progesterone and testosterone in conjunction with adrenaline. The sacral chakra governs relationships of all kinds which arise from the choices made through the energy of the solar plexus. It stimulates the continual changes that need to be made to create a productive environment in which they can be expressed. Change at its most creative arises through co-operation rather than coercion and comes through a willingness to adapt to what is required rather than a resistance to it which may result in having change forced upon us. The ability to change always begins with the relationship that we make with ourselves and which is reflected in all our other relationships.

7 Base Chakra

This can be explored as it articulates in the bones, muscles and joints of the skeleton with the flow of adrenaline that sustains movement in the physical body. The physical body is the most evident expression of the movement of energy through the other six chakras. When we are fully grounded in body our senses become wholly awake, so that we can really see what we are looking at, listen properly to what is being said, take time to think before speaking, smell deeply when inhaling, taste appreciatively when eating, feel what we are touching and concentrate when moving.

When the senses of the body are fully activated there is a return to the crown chakra to draw further inspiration for the faculties of the mind; thus the turning circle of the chakras is complete.

The following chapters in this section show how energy correlates with health through the senses of the body and faculties of the mind. A state of

Correlating energy with health

Aura	Chakra	Physical function	Healthcare	Mental correlative
Divine	Crown	Sensation	Assessing intelligence	Responding uniquely
Spirit	Brow	Adaptation	Understanding stress	Acting spontaneously
Soul	Throat	Respiration	Expressing energy	Seeking inspiration
Mind	Heart	Circulation	Allowing love	Inviting compassion
Astral	Solar plexus	Digestion	Nourishing well-being	Accepting responsibility
Etheric	Sacral	Regulation	Accepting change	Adapting freely
Physical	Base	Articulation	Exercising energy	Being grounded

well-being comes about when both are working efficiently and in harmony. Each chapter considers a specific physical process in the body and the accompanying psychological awareness required. Each one of the auric bodies represents a particular level of energy, from the most subtle to the most tangible.

The Divine energy is reflected through the crown chakra, which activates the functions of the brain and nervous system, manifesting as intelligence. This is expressed uniquely in every being because energy is in a new configuration at every instant: it cannot repeat itself but can only respond to conditions as they arise in the moment.

The Spirit energy is reflected through the brow chakra, which activates the functions of the endocrine system. They respond spontaneously to release the specific hormones that allow both body and mind to adapt to changing circumstances. This mirrors the human capacity to initiate actions that are informed by applying intelligence, so that we can respond most effectively to such changing circumstances.

The Soul energy is reflected through the throat chakra that activates the physical respiratory functions, the psychological correspondence of which is the process of inspiration, being inspired by fresh insights. Genuine inspiration carries a life force that revivifies the mind as oxygen revivifies the blood.

The Mind energy is reflected through the heart chakra which activates the heart and the circulation of the blood, carrying the life force throughout the whole system. Its psychological correlative is the experience of love that, at its most complete and expansive, affects the whole being. It is not confined, however, solely to the individual, because it has the capacity for a wider universal expression and that, when sought, manifests as compassion. This is generally recognized when it appears not only in the great spiritual teachers or humanitarians but also on an ordinary human level when people go beyond their limited desires in a commitment to serving others.

The Astral energy is reflected through the solar plexus chakra which activates everything that needs to be digested, both physically and psychologically. The process of digestion separates the pure from the impure, eliminating what may harm the body and utilizing what nourishes it. This process is automatic and involves no conscious choice. What we eat or drink, however, does involve choice and therefore responsibility. The psychological correlate of this is to take responsibility for our emotions and this involves a similar process of discernment, using what is beneficial and discarding what is harmful. With both we create nutritional stores which give us the finest and most suitable ingredients for living.

Taking responsibility focuses and concentrates energy rather than dispersing it, either through lack of attention or assigning responsibility for what happens to us elsewhere.

The Etheric energy is reflected through the sacral chakra which activates the regulatory systems so that they can maintain the life force in the body. The life force is contained within the system when all the structures and functions of the body and mind are able to support it; this requires the ability to respond swiftly and effectively to the ever-changing conditions which arise in both the external and internal environments. When there is resistance to change both the body and the mind can become constricted, slowing down the interactions throughout the energy field. When, however, there is an openness to change, all the levels of energy can come into alignment with one another so that the whole being becomes stabilized, allowing changes to take place without inhibition.

The Physical energy is reflected through the base chakra, which activates both movement and stillness in the physical body. There is no more evident and substantial expression of energy than that of the human form: it can convey information throughout every aspect of its being, in thoughts, words and actions. Being centred in mind is the mental correlative to being grounded in the body, allowing both to access strength from the earth. From this position both body and mind become ready and able to respond to change: to accept responsibility, to express love, to seek inspiration, to act spontaneously and above all to respond uniquely to life.

2.2

Energy through the Four Constitutions

I died as mineral and became a plant,
I died as a plant and rose to animal,
I died as animal and I was Man.

JALAL AL-DIN RUMI

Spiralling threads of energy manifest themselves in nature through every life form. Drawing on the elements of air, water, fire and earth, they adapt to the temperatures of cold, damp, heat and dryness around them, playing the roles that are necessary for their survival and exhibiting the characteristics that distinguish them from one another. At the centre of this continuous interplay of movement is the unique self, the identity of every being, which acts as the controller, responding to ongoing sensations and processing them so they can be seen and understood. It is through the complete self that consciousness finds its fullest expression, since this is the point of integration where the exterior conditions of interplay and delineation align with interior stillness and receptivity.

Energy through the four constitutions

Element	Humour	Temperament	Nature	Role	Character	Self
Air	Blood	Sanguine	Responsive	Interrogator	Perfectionist	Philosopher
Water	Phlegm	Phlegmatic	Sensitive	Victim	Martyr	Visionary
Fire	Yellow bile	Choleric	Active	Controller	Intimidator	Pioneer
Earth	Black bile	Melancholic	Receptive	Recluse	Rescuer	Peacemaker

2.3

Assessing Intelligence

As man thinketh in his heart, so God liveth
in the hollow of his heart, filling it with
immortality, light and intelligence.

THE VEDAS

On this plane of existence the mind expresses itself through the body and the soul, reflecting from one to the other the impressions it receives. The light of mind is ever present, its purpose to make sense of these impressions through the faculties of instinct, feeling, intellect, imagination and intuition. It is our senses that bring us to mind, offering a vast range of sensations to experience and explore. Through these we may identify with one another and form a collective consciousness, which brings ideologies such as religion and culture into being. Our minds may follow tracks which are similar to each other, but never identical. Just as there is no replication in nature, so there is no identification through comparison between one creature and another, for each being is unique in its essential composition.

True identification occurs through reconnection with the source of being, by the alignment of mind, body and soul, which act as channels to receive the light of consciousness. This identification with the source of being is the most precious gift of consciousness, given that it is the drawing close of the human to the divine; it is in 'minding our own business' that we are drawn back to this source.

Just as the body requires nourishment and care, so does the mind. Its faculties need to be developed and explored in all their forms. If the body is cared for at the expense of the mind, an imbalance occurs, but when both are attended to equally they work in harmony with one another, enabling them to develop their potential. The more we understand about the nature and meaning of intelligence, the greater the choice we have in how we use it; to dream through our lives or to wake up to our real selves.

Intelligence is frequently measured by academic prowess but there is an increasing awareness of the importance of other skills, such as the ability to recognize and express feelings, and to create and sustain satisfying relationships. The traditional perspective of intelligence as being based on rational and analytical skills needs to be reassessed. It covers a far wider spectrum, which includes physical, emotional and spiritual dimensions. Viewed from this perspective, intelligence becomes an unlimited force for growth, that finds itself at the heart of whatever matter is being addressed. This is a point of clarity, prior to the diversity and complexity which later emerges, and relates to the heart chakra which is the seat of consciousness. Knowledge in any form cannot in reality be deduced but only expressed when the heart is allowed its rightful place as the guiding light to the moment in all its potential, so that what is known is inspired through love.

The Four Elements as they Relate to the Crown Chakra

Energy rains down through the crown chakra into all the other chakras. The crown chakra's function is to make sense of the never-ending sensations which are experienced during life. This comes about through the interpretative skills of the brain, so that a unifying perspective is created, which allows intelligence to express itself.

There are four ways of expressing intelligence – through the body, feelings, intellect and soul – which are cultivated through the elements of air, water, fire and earth. Air is the origin of the breath and water of the form; fire maintains a working temperature and earth grounds it in a material world. The constitution of air is dynamic and infinite in its ability to inspire the life force, which is regulated through the water it absorbs. It is the heat of the fire that drives the water sufficiently so that it can settle in an earthly form, which takes the shape of a body in life, and ashes in death.

The four elements

Air
Water
Fire
Earth

These characteristics are applied in traditions such as

Assessing spiritual intelligence through the four elements as they relate to the crown chakra

Manifesting as: **Responding by:**

Air – intellectual intelligence through five faculties of the mind:

instinct	examining gut instincts
feelings	experiencing emotions
intellect	analysing events
imagination	picturing situations
intuition	trusting first thoughts

Water – emotional intelligence through five feelings:

grief/acceptance	acknowledging
fear/bravery	supporting
hate/love	allowing
anger/kindness	expressing
anxiety/empathy	investigating

Fire – spiritual intelligence through five capacities of the soul:

belief	committing
willingness	serving
acceptance	allowing
perseverance	enduring
truthfulness	integrating

Earth – physical intelligence through five senses of the body:

sound	listening
sight	observing
touch	massaging
taste	savouring
smell	absorbing

astrology and acupuncture. They may also be observed in everyday attitudes and behaviour, such as in the airy mind that darts from topic to topic; in the watery emotions that release intense feelings; in the fiery enthusiasm that can inflame new ventures; and in the earthly stability that maintains the routines and structures of life throughout the cycles of nature.

Elements relate to the sensations that are experienced instantaneously.

These sensations are activated through the nervous system which responds to them, so that the connection may be formulated between what has happened and how to react to it. When this link is established one is able to respond to oneself through the light of intelligence which illuminates the mind so that body can follow its instructions. Responding fully to oneself opens a gate in the mind to self-knowledge, the essential guide to being educated through life experience rather than intimidated by it.

The Seven Gates to Spiritual Perception

Within the context of the paradigm described in the table 'Energy through Light into Form' (see page 14) the seven gates of spiritual perception reflect the progression of pure light into the spectrum of colours, as seen for example in those of the rainbow.

Pure light reflects the finest, most elevated form of energy. As light slows down it descends into different colours, each of which has its own vibrational frequency and its own specific effects in the electromagnetic field of every being. The power of colour is both immediate and evocative in its impact: it has the ability to convey meaning in its most direct and specific form, both through visual impact and through the effect that it has throughout all the activities which take place in the electromagnetic spectrum of energy.

The seven gates to spiritual perception are opened through the light of understanding. We come to know ourselves most completely through spiritual intelligence, which enables us to differentiate between the state of being and the conditions of doing. The former centres and grounds us so that the mind, body and soul may come into alignment, and the latter moves us to assert ourselves, as we encounter life in its extensive range of possibilities. Spirit is life; when it withdraws from the body, it leaves an empty case. Whilst it is the breath of life, it does not define it. That is the work of the soul, which receives the effusion of the spirit, so that it many inspire the senses of the body through the faculties of the mind.

Spirit blows through the air, flows in the water, burns in life, and settles in the earth. Where there is life there is spirit, bringing everything into being.

Spiritual intelligence is innate in the nature of everything. It seeks to make the connection between the known and the unknown, so our lives have a purpose and meaning. Spiritual practices such as meditation and prayer are preparations to receive the light of consciousness as it manifests itself through each unique being, so that it may become wholly aware of itself. It does not come through duty or desire, but reveals itself when the conditions are right, that is when the energy of the heart has expanded to receive it in its full measure. Life experience which has accumulated memories of pain and difficulty may cause this energy to contract, constricting the ability to receive love and return it in compassion. It is only through the practice of loving-kindness both to oneself and others, that we may find the courage to allow the heart to open up to the divine beauty within the human condition. There is an important distinction between being kind and doing good: the former evolves naturally through feelings such as empathy and generosity, whilst the latter may be manipulated through wanting to prove one's own worth. It is only by being true to one's authentic self that one can discern the difference. This in itself is an ongoing process of discernment, because the authentic self is not fixed in its expression, but is continually evolving and refining according to the demands made of it and the truthful responses required by it. This process of refinement produces the key which opens the door to spiritual intelligence.

The seven gates to spiritual perception are listed below with their colours, openings and effects.

- White into purple – Seeking beauty which lifts the spirit.
- Indigo blue – Being generous which warms the soul.
- Turquoise – Encouraging compassion which opens the mind.
- Green – Expanding consciousness which develops the feelings.
- Yellow – Absorbing experiences which strengthen stamina.
- Orange – Being adaptable which instigates movement.
- Red – Staying grounded which encourages focus.

Expressive Statements

To speak assertively is to affirm one's own truth directly and with confidence. It does not use words as weapons of attack, either to injure or to manipulate communication, but as a means to express the reality of what the speaker wants to say. This form of speech may require preparation and practice before it becomes integrated into the way we express ourselves.

Expressive statements

Use the personal pronoun 'I'	I want you to clear up the mess in your room.
Avoid questions	Why can't you clear up all this mess?
Own your own responses	I don't like mess because …
Be specific	I want you to clear up the mess in your room today.
Keep on track	I appreciate how much you have to do but I want you to clear this mess because …
Broken record	Let's get back to what I was asking you to do …
Negotiation	Let's agree to a time when you can clean your room.
How to say 'no'	I don't want to go out today.
Be specific	I don't want to go out today because …
Show empathy	I really appreciate the work that you have done in arranging this.
Reject a request, not the person	I really enjoy your company, but I don't want to do this because …
Broken record	I have to say no again to your invitation because …
Avoid guilt	I'm really sorry to have to let you down.
Closure	I'm glad that's sorted out. Now …

Aggressive (attacking)	
Abusive	You really are so useless.
Blaming	It's all your fault.
Complaining	Why can't things be run properly?
Overreacting	Nothing will ever improve.

Indirect (hiding)	
Confusing	It might be like this, but it could be like that.
Guilt inducing	Why do you make me feel so unhappy?
Manipulative	If we spread a rumour about …
Sarcastic	Aren't you the clever one.

Passive (complaining)	
Apologetic	I'm only …
Indecisive	I want my life to change but nothing ever seems to happen.
Long-suffering	Why is life so cruel to me?
Negative	Everything I do goes wrong.

Assertive (enlightening)	
Direct	Let's look at what's really happening …
Open-minded	I hear what you say …
Respectful	I want to encourage us all to speak for ourselves …
Responsive	I want to help you to help yourself.

As children we may not have been listened to, or taken seriously, and this is often repeated in adulthood. Fear may be the key motivator which prevents us from expressing ourselves with honesty. When this situation arises we may feel that the only way we can be heard is to draw attention to ourselves either by prevarication, by taking on the role of a victim, through aggression or by withdrawing into deliberate non-communication.

We need to assess ourselves in our ability to be assertive. Are we able to:

- accept criticism,
- admit mistakes,
- ask for help,
- offer constructive criticism,
- deal with bureaucracy,
- explain feelings, and
- say no?

When we are able to achieve these targets we can learn to respect the influence of words and use them with care and economy so that the meaning is clearly expressed.

Healing Intelligence

The act of healing defines intelligence, by clearing blocked energy so that the light of consciousness shines with greater clarity. There is no energy without intelligence; it is innate within each pulse that animates life and in every cell of the body. It expresses itself through the nervous systems which enable communication to take place. At the heart of intelligence is the ability to sense one's own internal and external surroundings and to be able to respond to them appropriately. When there is a fluency between the systems of the mind and body, intelligence may be reflected in depth, so that one may engage in a relationship with oneself at a profound level, and which will be reflected in those around us.

Within this place of ease the mind becomes more focused, releasing memories, revealing insights and clarifying ideas. So often our minds respond to us as though we are flicking the channels on the remote control, producing a myriad of impressions, swiftly observed and easily forgotten. Yet whatever our thoughts may be, their function is to mirror the light of consciousness as it seeks to make itself known through us. The work of healing is based in consciousness. Since energy follows thought, how and what we think will affect the outcome of the treatment. Healing work embraces all aspects of intelligence. It encourages the practitioner to develop a relationship with their intelligence that is akin to that of a mystic; mindful of thoughts, yet not seeking to become entangled by them. Doing so engenders a clarity of mind in the practitioner upon which information from any of the seven levels of energy in the patient may be received, and imparted to them if appropriate, to illuminate understanding.

2.4

Understanding Stress

We are what we think.
All that we are arises with our thoughts.
With our thoughts we make the world.

GAUTAMA THE BUDDHA

Being stressed equates to being under pressure. Tension builds up in one part of the energy system at the expense of the others, causing an imbalance which, if left untreated, will eventually result in energy becoming blocked and ultimately breaking apart.

The adrenal glands release adrenaline, and then cortisone, in an attempt to disperse the compressed energy. Whilst the energy may achieve a state of parole, no long-term release is possible without attention given to the causes of the stressful condition. For full release to come about, self-knowledge is required. It is important to remember that ignorance of the self does not infer a lack of knowledge, but rather a turning away from it. Major contributions to stress are the expectations that we place on ourselves and on one another. Expectations create a gap between the reality of the present and the illusion of the future, leading to dissatisfaction with what we have and a yearning for what we don't. They carry with them an inbuilt assumption of their right to be fulfilled that generates frustration with life. In demanding rights we have to assert our will so that we can control the situation. The more we do so, motivated by notions of what we ought to be or have, the more the energy is directed towards desire. This focus on want disconnects us from being grounded in life. As time goes by our energy diminishes, trapped in a web of frustrated anticipation.

The antidote to stress is to step back from our wishes for the future and to reconsider the situations in which we find ourselves. When we do so, we may receive intuitive flashes of understanding, but often the process is more laborious, with time and space required for therapies, reflection, and sometimes medication (although with the latter preferably on a short-term basis). When we are stressed, we lose our sense of balance. We may feel separated from ourselves and from others, and thus need to reconnect to our own inner sense of being, and to the world around us. Everyone has to follow their own unique healing path and be willing to go wherever it leads. This requires commitment for a journey begun without any discernible end, although its aim – which is well-being – is attainable every step of the way.

The Four Humours as they Relate to the Brow Chakra

The brow chakra has an exterior aspect which relates to the appearance and movement of rational thought, and an interior aspect relating to the 'inner eye' of intuition and which can go beyond the sequential nature of rational thought to produce direct perception in the mind.

Element	Humour
Air	Blood
Water	Phlegm
Fire	Yellow bile
Earth	Black bile

The elements of air, water, fire and earth control the bodily humours or fluids of blood, phlegm, and yellow and black bile. Blood is generated through the oxygen carried in the air. Phlegm arises from the combination of water and air to stabilize the flow of fluid. Yellow bile, or bilirubin, comes from the breakdown of red blood cells. It contributes to the beginning of digestion by emulsifying fats so that they can be absorbed into the blood stream. Black bile deepens the colour and consolidates excreta, the waste products which are eliminated at the end of the process.

Within the context of ancient medicine the word humour relates to bodily fluids, but in modern times it is also used to describe the state of mind, such as when a person is bad-humoured, good-humoured, ill-humoured or when they have a good sense of humour.

* * *

Energy through the four humours

Air	Fire
Sanguine – responsive – absorbent	**Choleric** – activated – structured
Adaptable	Aggressive
Fleeting	Dramatic
Impatient	Extrovert
Irresponsible	Intolerant
Lively	Obstinate
Sociable	Pioneer
Industrious	Practical

Water	Earth
Phlegmatic – sensitive – patient	**Melancholic** – receptive – repetitive
Dreamy	Demanding
Passive	Gloomy
Persevering	Introspective
Relentless	Reserved
Shy	Retentive
Thoughtful	Sympathetic
Pragmatic	Diligent

All four humours interact with one another on a continuous basis in order to maintain a stability which can sustain the life force. When there is an excess of one humour there will be a deficiency in another, followed by sympathetic responses from the other two. An excess of air creates a strong wind, which may manifest itself in turbulent states of mind or in irregular circulation of the blood. Overflowing water produces a swamp, which reveals itself in lachrymose states of mind and respiratory illnesses ranging from colds to pneumonia. Too much fire generates rage in the mind and burning in the body, particularly in the stomach and small intestine, resulting in ulcers and liver disorders. An excess of earth causes energy to stagnate so that the mind becomes fixed and the body turgid with undigested matter, as seen in conditions such as depression and constipation.

Imbalance amidst the fluids of the body puts it into a state of distress, which is reflected by the condition of the mind. Stress builds up when the tension it creates cannot be released because its source remains hidden from view. Once revealed, it allows solutions to emerge which may allow an ease of movement through both mind and body. When the energy in the humours is allowed to move freely along its appointed directions it responds spontaneously to both the internal conditions of the body and the external surroundings of

Understanding stress through the four humours as they relate to the brow chakra

Manifesting as:	Expressing by:	Manifesting as:	Expressing by:
	Air – blood		**Fire – yellow bile**
irrationality	encouraging left-brain activities	impatience	setting realistic targets
indecisiveness	developing intuition	intolerance	examining attitudes
preoccupiation	allocating time for specific tasks	addiction	examining underlying emotions
restlessness	re-evaluating needs	impulsiveness	learning from past actions
	Water – phlegm		**Earth – black bile**
anxiousness	seeking cognitive or psychotherapy	withdrawal	seeking some company every day
clumsyness	practising grounding exercises	depression	taking exercise
moodyness	opening up to distress	ritualistic behaviour	doing something new regularly
weepyness	allowing release of grief	feeling drained	arranging regular periods of relaxation

nature, interacting between the two so that they are as a mutual support for one another.

The Seven Levels of the Accumulation of Stress

Within the context of the paradigm which is described in the table 'Energy through Light into Form' on page 14 the seven levels of accumulation of stress are reflected in the seven layers of the aura revealing what is happening through the seven levels of energy in a continual moving picture show composed of blocks of colour and shifting images. They represent what is happening in the present and what has happened in the past, through the shapes and intensity of colour at each level which reflect the impact of life experience throughout the energy field. The levels of stress associated with each level of the aura are as follows:

Physical: carried through the bloodstream and lodged in the physical structures and functions of the body when tensions cannot be released.

Etheric: acquired from the planes of existence prior to conception and through genetic inheritance.

Astral: absorbed through the intensity of unresolved emotional experiences, dating back from memories

	which have been transmitted through the generations into present time.
Mind:	held in the instincts, feelings, intellect and imagination and freed through the intuition when the constriction of negative thought gives way to the possibility of positive outcomes.
Soul:	covered over with the pressure of unprocessed pain, creating the states of depression, neurosis and personality disorders.
Spirit:	darkened by the disconnection from the realities of life, developing into conditions of acute or chronic psychosis.
Divine:	prevented from connecting to the spiritual nature through the accumulation of unprocessed experiences stored in the other six levels of energy.

To find out how we accumulate stress we need to uncover the cause. By observing the interplay between the elements and fluids which sustain our essential composition, we can learn how the humours manifest in ourselves, so that we can observe any imbalance. When air meets water it bubbles up; if there is too much it disperses widely. Too much air at a high altitude thins the blood; too much water saturates it. When water meets fire it cools it down, but too high a temperature evaporates it. When air meets earth it can lift it up; too much air may cause turbulence; too little deprives it of the carbon dioxide and oxygen essential for breath. When earth meets fire it can be heated up. Too many flames will scorch it; too few will cause it to become cold and dense, as solid as frozen mud.

These permutations between elements and humours occur in us as well as in nature, since it supports all our body processes. By observing the qualities of the elements and humours, and how they affect both ourselves and others, we may begin to gain insight into them and how they react to one another.

People of a blood humour predominately come under the element of air. Ideas fly into their minds continually, so frequently that they may become 'light-headed' and need to find ways to ground themselves through practical activities.

For those of a phlegm humour water predominates. They may feel internally dehydrated and need to absorb water in great amounts, not only by drinking but also through such activities as water sports. Sharing the depth of their feelings is also essential for them.

Those who are predominately of a yellow bile humour are ruled by fire which can cause them to become 'hot-headed'. Impulsive and quick to anger, they may need cooling water to quench their ardour and a lightness of touch to provide a calming influence.

Those of a predominately black bile humour come under the element of earth. They may become entrenched in their habits, 'stick-in-the-muds' unable to adapt or change easily because they are overly dependent on routines which shore up an underlying sense of insecurity. They need the elements of water to free them from the earth, air to inspire them and fire to encourage them.

When there is an excess of air in the mind, thoughts can arise like a whirlwind, flying off in every direction with nothing strong enough to ground them. It can become difficult to access the other faculties of consciousness, such as feelings, imagination and intuition. The antidote to such a condition is to become more grounded, spending some time in reflection or meditation, or in carrying out straightforward practical tasks such as cooking, cleaning or gardening. This enables thoughts to become focused in everyday living and gives a 'breathing space' to the workings of the rational mind.

When there is an excess of water in the mind, feelings can become over-whelming, drowning out rational or creative thought processes. In order to balance this torrential flow of water some of it needs to be drained out, to allow air to circulate and refresh the rational mind. One way in which this can happen is not to stem any tears which may arise, but to allow them full flow. Another antidote to this condition is to exercise reason in the form of active listening, by providing a reflective setting in which the speaker may come to understand the underlying reasons for emotional turmoil.

When there is an excess of fire in the thought processes it can stimulate the production of yellow bile, creating a bilious state of mind, which has a tendency to meet situations with a backlog of unresolved and therefore toxic anger. Such flames of rage can be cooled down by calming the fiery mind with subtle and sensitive listening and by redirecting the energetic power of anger into work which is both innovative and challenging.

When there is an excess of earth in a mental state it can bring about a fixed state of mind, which clings to attitudes and habits, creating attachments that are highly resistant to any form of change. The antidote to this state of mind is to introduce change very slowly and gently, allowing the cycles of both thoughts and events to unfold organically, without any interference or imposition but with encouragement and practical guidance.

Thinking, feeling, acting and reacting are all fundamental aspects of our nature and conditioning, arising from the functioning of the four elements. The more we understand why we think, feel, act and react the way we do, the more able we will be to respond to stressful situations and find our own ways of resolving them.

To understand the origin of stress it can be helpful to evaluate your state of health in relation to your physical, psychological and spiritual needs:

Understanding stress questionnaire

Symptom	Never	Rarely	Occasionally	Frequently
Physical				
Headaches				
Skin rashes				
Sore throats/colds				
Digestive problems				
Low libido				
Spinal problems				
Clumsy/accident prone				
Psychological				
Anxious				
Tearful				
Irritable				
Indecisive				
Irrational				
Mood swings				
Depressed				
Spiritual				
Destructive habits				
Inflexible beliefs				
Apathetic				
Sleep problems				
Inability to concentrate				
Loss of interest				
Disconnection from daily life				

Expressive Listening

The pressure of feeling stressed can be released greatly by talking to someone who is a willing listener. In the space that is created through listening there is time not only to hear the words spoken but also the meanings that lie beyond them. Words define the feelings, the thoughts, the images and the instincts that arise in our mind. When these experiences are shared they are like a two-way mirror, reflecting back to us in all their potential to explain, to enlighten and to educate. Listening skills lie at the heart of all creative relationships. The more we listen to one another, the more we may be able to share, to empathize and to identify our common needs.

Barriers to Hearing

◆ Not allowing sufficient time to give oneself fully to the act of listening ('I must leave soon, I've got too much to do …').

◆ Becoming distracted by the surroundings, e.g. books on shelves, pictures on walls, layout of furniture, noise outside …

◆ Thinking about something else instead of listening to the speaker ('I wonder if I have enough time to arrange …').

◆ Reacting to the speaker's words as though they were a personal affront ('How can he/she speak like that about …?').

◆ Losing the thread of the conversation ('I'm getting so confused by all these details …').

◆ Preventing the speaker from completing what needs to be said ('Oh, I know what you mean, when I …').

◆ Giving oneself responsibility for having to solve the speaker's problems ('Now, if I were you, I would …').

Hearing what is spoken is of inestimable value, because it creates an intimacy, which is a conduit to closeness, allowing confidences to be shared and problems to be resolved through mutual support.

Gateways to Hearing

◆ Be generous with your time: make it freely available for as long as seems appropriate.

- Be settled and comfortable so that you will not become restless and distract the speaker.

- Be willing to be a mirror to the speaker's words so that the speaker can hear them more clearly.

- Be open to the words but don't demand a meaning: allow it to unfold as it wills.

- Be non-judgemental and non-attached to the thoughts and opinions of the speaker: they belong to the speaker and not to you.

- Be patient: don't interrupt unless absolutely necessary because it may block the unfoldment of what the speaker needs to express.

- Be free of the desire to solve any problems: they are not yours to solve; your responsibility is to be with the person as they work through their conflict.

Healing Stress

The act of healing provides release from stress and may even induce in the patient a state of peacefulness hitherto unknown. This can be a revelation, freeing the patient from the burdens of inner and outer conflict. In dealing with stress we accept the source of tension for what it is, and seek to effect change through reflecting on it rather than reacting to it. It is not a denial of the tensions inherent in everyday life but a decision to meet life as it really is – in us and as it is mirrored in the world around us.

Healing work can reduce or even dissolve the effects of stress by helping patients to get to the root of their problems. It can reconnect patients to their inner resources. These are most directly accessed by accepting fully the present state and being prepared to work with it without any recrimination or blame. This helps patients to remain centered in their own being without becoming involved in the lives of others at the expense of their own needs.

2.5

Expressing Energy

Speak what we feel, not what we ought to say.

WILLIAM SHAKESPEARE, *KING LEAR*

There is no life without expression, since it gives voice to the energy of consciousness. Everything in life creates its own sound and expresses itself in its own unique way. The earth's atmosphere communicates through the rain and wind. Other voices, such as plants, are less obvious, however, through attunement with their energy we can hear them. Such attunement is already practised with animals, for example by horse whisperers. Of all the voices of energy, the human one carries the greatest range of meaning. It carries with it the potential for both good and harm in the use of words. We need, therefore, to remember to speak consciously as much as possible and to refrain from the negative aspects of careless speech such as speaking ill of others, betraying confidences, spreading rumours and judging others through habitual criticism.

The Four Temperaments as they Relate to the Throat Chakra

The throat chakra inspires expression in every form, giving voice to all the sounds of creation. Seeking to express one's own truth lies at the heart of all genuine communication and observing how one speaks with others may help us to do this. Studying the four temperaments shows us why conversations can blow hot or cold, why some expressions are wet and why humour can be dry. The four temperaments derive their nature from the four temperatures of dry, wet, hot and cold, which affect both the internal and external environment of the body.

There are a number of factors that affect the climate within the body and mind, such as the weather. Wind can be bracing or calming; rain can be

Element	Humour	Temperament
Air	Blood	Sanguine
Water	Phlegm	Phlegmatic
Fire	Yellow bile	Choleric
Earth	Black bile	Melancholic

refreshing or debilitating; heat can be invigorating or relaxing; dampness can be soothing or uncomfortable. All these temperatures affect the ability of both the body and the mind to adapt to changing circumstances, both outside and inside the system.

Another factor causing climate change within the body and the mind is the food or drink that we take in. Most fruits and vegetables have a cooling effect, whilst dairy products, meat, poultry and fish generate warmth in the internal environment. Sugars, sweets and fried foods create heat and damp; alcohol and spicy foods cause heat and wetness. Avocados, bananas, raw foods and ice cream bring about cold and damp; dairy produce and cold foods generate coldness and wetness. It is useful to consider the impact of food and drink on the body temperature so that it can be maintained at a level which supports the smooth running of the structures and functions of the body and the faculties of the mind.

A third factor affecting the personal climate is the atmosphere that is absorbed in daily life. A 'chilly' atmosphere can create feelings of discomfort and even fear; a cold atmosphere can be unwelcoming and even hostile; a 'frozen' atmosphere can be challenging and unproductive, whilst a warm atmosphere conveys the presence of friendliness and hospitality. There is often an instinctive response to the temperature in the setting created by others, which influences how we respond to them

A fourth factor that influences the internal and external environment of the body is geographical location: the thinner the atmosphere, the harder it is to breathe; the presence of lakes, rivers and the sea can be both calming and reflective; crowded towns and cities can feel exhilarating in the presence of so much activity or overwhelming in their intrusion on personal space; large tracts of isolated land can seem disturbing because of the lack of human contact or restorative to those who seek seclusion.

Whilst the internal climate is composed of all four conditions, hot, cold, wet and dry, one temperament appears in the ascendant at any one time and may be clearly seen, whilst the second appears in the descendant, partially or deeply hidden from view. The other two may be even more deeply hidden but can appear when they are needed, such as in a time of crisis. For example the fire energy of a fever is generated to destroy harmful microorganisms; the water energy of excessive sweat releases excess fluid from the body to re-establish the electrolyte balance; the air energy in excessive flatulence helps to release pressure which has built up in the abdomen; the earth energy creates faeces to eliminate toxins.

The climate of the sanguine temperament comes about through the interaction between the element of air and the humour of blood. It can have a 'lively' presence and be detected in those with a ruddy complexion. The sanguine temperament can be as cool as air, quick to respond and easily deflected, like the wind as it changes direction. This temperament thrives on stimulus, reacting swiftly to the moment. As it is already flexible in mind it often needs to become more focused in body, to pit its wits against something, so that ideas may be grounded in action. In order to create a more productive environment it may need to draw first on the warmth and enthusiasm of the choleric humour to expand its vision and then to absorb the cool receptivity of the phlegmatic humour to deepen it. This sanguine temperament may be light-headed in the way that it expresses itself; it often needs to be grounded through analytical thought so that it can make the best use of the inspirations which arise with such frequency and ease.

The climate of the phlegmatic temperament comes about through the interaction between the element of water and the humour of phlegm. It can have a sensitive presence and be seen in those who have a translucent complexion. The phlegmatic temperament can be super absorbent, soaking up water continually and, chameleon-like, ever changing to blend in with its environment. This temperament relates to deeply felt emotions, which act as a driving force to uncover the feelings that lie hidden within them, waiting to reveal their underlying truth. In order to create a more understanding environment the phlegmatic temperament needs to draw upon the reflective characteristics of the element of earth, so that feelings may be reflected upon rather than acted out. Once understood, the element of air can enlighten them and that of fire put them in a more expansive context, so that when integrated this temperament can also support others in their quest for emotional understanding.

The climate of the choleric temperament evolves through the interaction between the element of fire and the humour of yellow bile. It can have a bold presence and can be seen in those with a flushed complexion. The choleric temperament can be as combustible as a forest fire. It can blaze in anger, permeating rage as it spreads itself and needs a natural firewall to contain it so that it may be directed into energy which can implement creative and constructive change. In order to create a more constructive environment the choleric temperament may draw upon the element of water to cool the flames with understanding, earth to calm them down and then air when ready to rise again to bring fresh inspiration.

The climate of the melancholic temperament evolves through the interaction between the element of earth and the humour of black bile. It can have a subdued presence and be observed in a sallow complexion. It can retreat into the dark of the underground until it is ready to face the light of day. This temperament relates to the element of earth and its cycles of growth, maturation, decay and renewal which maintain the whole of creation. It responds to the rhythms of nature, which it seeks to reflect in its own life. In order to create a more confident environment it needs to absorb water, so that it can soften and open up to the light. Unreleased emotions obscure the light of understanding but when they are set free they illuminate the darkened earth. Once the earth is softened it may gather the energies of air for breath and fire for warmth, so that it may become ground which can be fully cultivated for the production of all that is nourishing in life.

When there is an excessive predominance of one temperament at the expense of the others it can result in a fixity that inhibits freedom of expression. Inspiring ideas that emerge through the sanguine temperament have to be grounded to be fully realized; the deep feelings that come to the surface in the phlegmatic temperament need to be expressed rather than acted out; the fiery rages of the choleric temperament need to be tempered with self-reflection; the withdrawn states of the melancholic temperament have to be accepted and supported through sensitive and gentle encouragement into a more sociable context. Although these temperaments configure one at a time they need to be able to communicate with one another so that they can make the necessary adjustments in temperature which allow them to work together in the spirit of co-operation, to give expression to every state of being.

Energy through the four temperaments as they relate to the throat chakra

Manifesting as:	Expressing by:	Manifesting as:	Expressing by:
Air – sanguine		**Fire – choleric**	
blowing ideas in the air	allowing time for them to settle	dominating discussions	allowing others to speak
lacking focus in speech	observing the effect on the listener	very forceful in speech	letting others finish their speech
easily distracted	using 'broken record' technique to refocus	leading conversations	encouraging 'brainstorming' sessions
being 'high'-minded	encouraging a 'grounded' perspective	being tactless	thinking before speaking
Water – phlegmatic		**Earth – melancholic**	
absorbing emotions	speaking or writing about them	refraining from conversation	rehearsing communication skills
being overwhelmed by feelings	allowing time for reflection	repeating words	listening while speaking
creating dramas	considering the roles played by others	speaking slowly	watching the body language
being oversensitive	looking at the needs of the inner child	speaking despondently	observing how the listener responds

The voice of each of the four temperaments is highly distinctive. The sanguine sound has a shouting tone, as though it needs to be heard through high winds in its urgency to declare its thoughts. It can be difficult to follow since it may be attempting to communicate a number of ideas at the same time. When this energy is depleted it diminishes to a whisper, hesitant in what it wants to say because it is doubtful of the outcome. At its best, it carries well, and is the voice of the skilled negotiator, since it has a strong capacity for rational thought.

The phlegmatic voice may have groaning undercurrents as if weighed down by the sadness of life. It thrives on communication since it longs to be heard and will go to great lengths to draw attention to itself, sometimes through melodramatic and destructive forms of behaviour. On occasion it can have a pleading quality, when its energy is drained through tension. If problems are resolved it becomes soothing, taking on a mellifluous quality that can reassure those who hear it. This is the voice of the therapist, whose words are given to support others, so that their minds may be calmed.

The choleric voice holds laughter in its sound, responding to humour with enthusiasm and creating warmth in its tone. It may be become strident in battle and faulting in defeat, but in its mid-range is welcoming in the way it greets others. This is the voice of the performer who can command attention and hold it for sustained periods of time. In heated debate it can overrule others, with forceful opinions, as well as disarm, charming them with a ready wit, so that they melt into agreement.

The melancholic voice has a bell-like tone that often indicates a great facility for singing. It has a sympathetic resonance which attracts people who need help but who are unable to help themselves. As the voice of the musician it is able to carry the mind into memories and sensations that words cannot reach. It is easily dampened by disapproval, that controlling attitude which seeks to suppress or subjugate others. When there is appreciation and gratitude it grows in confidence, so that it is able to express itself in its own musical sound.

Within the context of the paradigm which is described in the table 'Energy through Light into Form' on page 14 the seven voices of expressive communication are activated by the seven chakras, the vortices of energy which set all the bodily and mental processes in motion. There is a level of existence where all things have speech and communication, one with the other. Expressive communication takes place in all seven levels of the energy field through the senses of the body and the faculties of the mind, when they are heard. This communication happens when there are no impediments to the flow of energy between each level.

The way we use our voices, and what we say, sets the tone for the dialogues that we have both with ourselves and one another. If we employ words to

The Seven Voices Of Expressive Communication

Chakra	Communication	Form
Crown	Expressive statements	How to speak for yourself
Brow	Expressive listening	How to hear
Throat	Expressive questions	How to keep your thoughts on track
Heart	Expressive bodies	How your mind uses your body to describe illness
Solar plexus	Expressive phrases	How your body describes its state of health
Sacral	Expressive muscles	How your muscles adapt to your mind
Base	Expressive actions	How your body reveals how you are

condemn, we stifle communication. When we make disparaging comments about others these may reflect how we really feel about ourselves. A constant need to be in the right may be due to having been made to feel in the wrong on a regular basis. Words always create an effect, sometimes long after they've been spoken. In order to have meaningful dialogues we need to be able to formulate questions that direct the flow of conversation.

Expressive Questions

These relate directly to what is being said so that the speaker can follow the thread of their own thoughts, without being distracted by the listener in any way. At their best, they need to be kept as brief as possible, so that the emphasis remains with the speaker rather than the listener.

Establish objectives:	'So what do you feel you want from this session?'
Avoid closed questions:	'Did that situation make you feel very unhappy?'
Ask open questions:	'How did you feel when that happened to you?'
Use playback:	'So when this happened to you, you felt very angry because …?'
Summarize:	'Are you feeling clearer about what has happened?'
Brainstorm:	'So how do you want to go forward from all this?'
	'Let's look at your options.'
Evaluate objectives:	'How are you feeling now?'
	'Do you feel that you need more support?'

By following this sequence the speaker is able to uncover what lies at the heart of whatever needs to be said. Listening wholeheartedly will enable the hearer to frame the questions through the content of the conversation. It will indicate what needs to be left alone and what needs to be followed through. Asking pertinent questions shows that we are really listening and helps to give the speaker the confidence to communicate from the heart.

Healing Communication

The act of healing communicates the language of energy, seeing it through the body and hearing it through the mind. In healing, communication is opened up at every level of energy, creating a relationship between the practitioner and patient that determines whether communication is whole or partial. If only partially transmitted, it is selective according to what the participants want to say and hear. If it is whole, however, in the spirit of attunement, it brings about an intimacy because of the lack of barriers to what may be shared. Intimacy cannot be forced but may be encouraged so that it becomes possible in every dialogue. Attunement to one another allows communication to serve its purpose, which is to enable life to make itself known, educating us through all the experiences of our lives, and drawing from us innate wisdom and authentic response.

2.6

Allowing Love

I follow the religion of love.
Whatever way love's mounts take,
that is my religion and faith.

MUHYIDDIN IBN 'ARABI, *TARJUMAN AL-ASHWAQ 11:15*

Allowing love into our lives is an act of faith. It cannot be seen or measured but only experienced in a way that is unique to every being. When love appears in our lives it 'softens' the heart so that energy can circulate more freely throughout all the systems. The feeling of love creates the willingness to co-operate with oneself, with others, and with life in general. When we come together in the acceptance of love, rather than the separation of conflict, we can explore the differences which divide us and look for the solutions that unite us. This is a process that requires compassion, so that it is possible to go beyond misunderstanding and allow forgiveness, firstly for oneself where one has caused harm, either to oneself or to others, and subsequently for others who may have harmed one, either subconsciously or with full intent. When we allow ourselves to be guided by love, it may transform our lives. Habitual patterns of constriction, negativity and fear may be transmuted into acceptance, allowing an understanding to emerge that helps us to make the choices that are right for us.

The Four Natures as They Relate to the Heart Chakra

The sensation of love arises through the heart chakra which is situated at the midpoint of the chest. It can give us the confidence

Element	Humour	Temperament	Nature
Air	Blood	Sanguine	Responsive
Water	Phlegm	Phlegmatic	Sensitive
Fire	Yellow bile	Choleric	Active
Earth	Black bile	Melancholic	Receptive

to find out about ourselves through our natures and how we apply them in our life experiences. There are four fundamental natures which are reflected in the four functions of the brain. The propensity to respond arises in the right frontal area. This is the nature of the explorer who loves to travel to new lands, in mind and body, and who hates to be trapped by regular routines and mundane events. The capacity to be sensitive emerges in the right basal function of the brain. This is the nature of the dramatist, who thrives on crises, real or perceived, which can be played out in a theatrical turn of events and whose senses would be dulled by an overly peaceful life. The power to be active appears in the left frontal section of the brain. This is the nature of the leader who likes to take charge and direct events and whose initiative is thwarted when not fully engaged in the thick of the action. The predisposition to be receptive unfolds through the left basal function of the brain. This is the nature of the recluse, who chooses solitude, preferring to focus energy on concentration and reflection.

Figure 25: How the brain works in relation to the four natures

Left frontal

Logic – leadership

I enjoy mathematics

I can make and mend machinery

I use computers and other forms of technology

I measure results through scientific proof

I am skilful with money

I am an effective problem-solver

I enjoy being in charge

Right frontal

Ideas – creativity

I often have new ideas

I like to work on several ideas together

I am very artistic

I have good hand-eye co-ordination

I have a good eye and sense of order

I have a good sense of humour

I prefer the large view to the detail

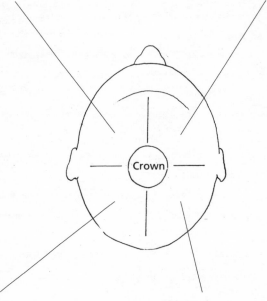

Left basal

Organization – routine

I am very well-organized

I enjoy detailed work

I prefer instructions to being left on my own

I am very loyal and reliable

I am very uncomfortable with disorder

I am very uncomfortable with emotional behaviour

I uphold traditional values

Right basal

Intuition – emotions

I am very intuitive

I am good at encouraging enthusiasm

I value relationships above worthy causes

I enjoy the creative arts

I am uncomfortable with conflict

I am easily moved to tears

I believe that the spiritual nature governs the
material world

Love through the four natures as they relate to the heart chakra

Manifesting as:	Allowing by:	Manifesting as:	Allowing by:
Air – responsive		**Fire – active**	
noncommittal	letting arrangements flow	impatient	slowing down body movements
abstracted	suggesting practical activities		
elusive	maintaining independent interests	intolerant	acknowledging each unique perspective
restless	providing a selection of options	controlling	concentrating on oneself
		impulsive	allowing time to make plans
Water – sensitive		**Earth – receptive**	
dependent	listening to underlying messages	moody	relating to the person, not to their state
melodramatic	recognizing but not engaging in the state	reserved	negotiating social arrangements in agreement
sociable	encouraging companionship	slow	being patient
intense	letting it flow to its natural conclusion	anxious	encouraging mental healthcare

Everyone has access to all these natures and to the potential contained within them. No one is fixed by a specific nature, but they are qualified by them, both through essential inclination and personal preference. When all of the natures are in harmony with one another they create the conditions for co-operation which are reflected throughout the whole energy field, allowing a natural order to unfold. At the heart of this co-operation is the acceptance of oneself, including one's faults; this can reveal the tendencies within one's nature and how to work with them towards greater self-awareness.

The Seven Keys to Heart-to-Heart Relationships

Within the context of the paradigm which is shown in the table 'Energy through Light into Form' on page 14 the seven keys to heart-to-heart relationships are transported along the pathways that direct energy from the chakras through the meridians into the physical organs of the body. Exploring the relationship between the meridians and the effects they have on both body and mind can show how they act as keys to understanding what inspires us and what holds us back. Each key opens the heart to a different expression of love from its effect on the physical body, which can be strengthened and given 'backbone', as reflected in the function of the governor vessel and from the experience of heartfelt emotions as reflected in the function of the conception vessel.

The lung and large intestine meridians are channels for the inspiration of love and for its purification; the stomach and spleen meridians are channels through which love can be absorbed and returned to its source. The heart and small intestine meridians carry the vitality of love, so that it can nourish the being in body, mind and soul. The bladder and kidney meridians transmit the sensations of love so that fear can be resolved. The pericardium and triple heater meridians transmit the protection and warmth that is necessary to preserve and maintain the love of life in every form. The gall bladder and liver meridians transmit energy for both planning and implementing activities, so that loving relationships can find new and creative ways of fulfilment.

Each meridian plays its part in channelling loving thoughts and sensations throughout the system to the relevant organs so that feeling may also be transmuted into action. For example, a feeling may result in a physical embrace, a sentiment may become expressed in words, music or art, and a philanthropic vision may be translated into projects of tangible help for those in need.

The real ground of all relationships is love, whether one is aware of it or not. It expresses itself in many forms including those of friendship, sexual attraction and family connections. The master key which opens the heart to real relationships is complete acceptance, without hierarchy. This gives us the freedom to express ourselves, to affirm our love and commitment, together with the trust to follow the feelings of attraction that motivated us in the first place.

Complete acceptance encourages us to learn about one another and to develop relationships which are creative and can adapt to new circumstances. Relationships are strengthened rather than diminished by problems or

The seven keys to heart-to-heart relationships

Heart setting	Meridian
Heartened by the physical proximity of the two vessels	Governor & conception vessels Spleen & stomach Kidney & bladder Liver & gall bladder
Drawn together through the power of electromagnetism	Governor & conception vessels Spleen & stomach Kidney & bladder Liver & gall bladder
Not only survive conflicts but are strengthened by them	Governor & conception vessels Stomach & spleen Kidney & bladder Liver & gall bladder
Based on equality in relationship to one another	Governor & conception vessels Lung & large intestine Spleen & stomach Heart & small intestine Kidney & bladder Triple heater & heart protector Gall bladder & liver
Change with the times but remain timeless in nature	Governor & conception vessel Large intestine & lung Stomach & spleen Bladder & kidney Triple heater & heart protector
Adapt to one another together through changing circumstances	Governor vessel Stomach & spleen Bladder & kidney Gall bladder & liver
Create the 'feelgood' factor	Governor vessel Bladder & kidney Gall bladder & liver

difficulties. Heart-to-heart relationships can stand the test of time; there is a spontaneous connection which can be reignited after separation, however long that period might be. These are relationships that generate a real pleasure in the company of one another; we are revived by them because they fulfil us, making the presence of love a reality in our lives.

The movement of love is circular. It begins in and returns to each self as it is experienced in every life. Love is ever present in the heart of every being, known or not.

Learning about the four natures can help us to understand our motives and behaviour in an expansive context so that we can recognize them and, where necessary, amend our thoughts and actions accordingly. It can also enable us to find more effective ways of co-operating with one another, so that misunderstandings and conflicts may be avoided through mutual tolerance and support.

The responsive nature is primarily peaceful, sanguine in temperament as it seeks the balance between being hot- or cold-blooded. Its aim is harmony in all things, and it explores many ways to bring this about. Ever ready to respond, it may be easily deflected but swiftly brought back into focus with the light touch of reason that grounds ideas into form. This nature respects the power of analytical thought and seeks proof to confirm its findings. It lends itself to mental stimulation and can be intolerant of instinctive and intuitive inspiration. It may seek the order of perfected thought, becoming frustrated when it is elusive. When this nature allows the other faculties of consciousness their rightful place amongst the functions of the mind, they enrich the whole perspective, bringing with them a depth of range and understanding that can only strengthen the peaceful accord that is so fundamental in this nature.

The sensitive nature is primordially passionate, phlegmatic in temperament, in that it ebbs and flows through the currents of life. It craves to be understood and will use any means at its disposal to make its feelings known. It experiences life with such intensity that it can appear to be drowning in the depths of its own emotions. It has an acute sense of its own feelings and also those of others. When feelings of emotional pain accumulate, this nature may seek release in alcohol or other drugs which may give effective, albeit temporary, relief. This is a nature that easily takes offence, especially when it receives unsolicited advice. Such sensitivity often puts it into conflict with others. It can be confrontational, provoking intense reactions. Although this nature can disrupt peace and create turmoil, it has an underlying drive to seek truth.

The active nature, which is choleric in humour, is fundamentally benevolent. It may be a joy to encounter unless it becomes overpowering. It is a nature that seeks a mission so that it can be fully employed, ensuring that its vibrant energy is not wasted in activities that have no goals, or misdirected with excessive zeal into leadership that has scant regard for its followers. When in balance this is the nature of the natural leader who takes others into battle, courageous in action and considerate to those who follow. This is a fiery nature, but when the flames are weak the joy of life dissipates. One of the causes of this depletion is losing face in the company of others when errors of leadership are revealed publicly. Just as it benefits from tactful and discreet correction, so it needs to assimilate these qualities in balancing its own natural enthusiasms.

The receptive nature, which is melancholic in temperament, is basically sympathetic. It absorbs atmosphere, assimilating feelings and seeking to nurture those in distress. Often it goes to extremes in taking on the burdens of others, shouldering them until they become so heavy that illness or injury can result. It can become so entangled in the affairs of others that the only antidote is to seek a place of retreat until it regains a sense of its own self. It may even become so depleted that it requires prolonged periods of rest to recover. Before it can be of effective help it needs to become more receptive to its own needs. Through reflection it learns to see where natural boundaries have to be drawn so that its innate tendency to sympathize does not allow its own energy to be misappropriated by those in need. When personal energy is drawn into others it weakens the boundaries between individuals and can make it unclear as to where responsibilities belong. There needs to be a balance between self-care and looking after others that enables the receptive nature to nurture both and not be drained in the process. This nature can offer the most productive support to those in need provided that it is receptive to the needs of it own being.

All the natures interact with one another so that they can fulfil their essential purpose, which is to complement one another rather than for one to dominate at the expense of the others. The earthly form provides a place of reflection for transcendent energy, so that it may reveal itself in the nature of every being.

Expressive Bodies

Every part of the body expresses its own nature. Each external form conveys an internal meaning, which helps us to understand what purpose it serves and what to investigate when there is any dysfunction. The relationships are listed below.

Every part of the body expresses intelligence. When information is received through the body parts it helps its owner to develop an understanding of why an illness or accident has happened. From the holistic perspective the body is the real measure of the state of health. It cannot lie; it is true to itself at every moment,

The relationships of the parts of the body

Blood	Life force	Large intestine	Acquisition
Skin	Barrier	Anus	Waste ground
Hair	Strength	Bones	Structure
Eyes	Insight	Back	Support
Ears	Obedience	Limbs	Mobility
Nose	Sniffing out	Muscles	Tensions
Mouth	Opening up	Joints	Flexibility
Teeth	Decisions	Shoulders	Responsibility
Chin	Holding up	Arms	Distance
Neck	Flexibility	Elbows	Direction
Throat	Communication	Hands	Holding
Lungs	Inspiration	Wrists	Restriction
Heart	Love	Fingers	Fine focus
Stomach	Holding in	Fingernails	Fine protection
Small intestine	Absorption	Hips	Balance
Liver	Organization	Legs	Striding out
Gall bladder	Frustration	Knees	Submission
Kidneys	Relationships	Ankles	Holding up
Bladder	Pressure	Feet	Stability
Vagina	Surrender	Toes	Dense focus
Penis	Power	Toenails	Dense protection

expressing unequivocally how it feels and thinks, and directing attention to where help is required. When we connect to what our physical body is saying about us we open up to the deeper levels of energy, allowing their innate intelligence, which is present by the very nature of their being, to make itself known.

Healing Love

The act of healing encourages love to fulfil the heart. Love's presence can be buried under layers of painful experiences which may not have been resolved. Stored pain may crystallize around the parts of the body where it was felt, creating a resistance to love. However, when the energy field becomes relaxed in a safe setting it allows love to be released. It follows the path of least resistance through the feeling of joy that it engenders. It seeks a relationship through which it can be channelled without constriction. The experience of love invites compassion so that how we feel is integrated into how we act both inwardly and outwardly. Compassion arises when love becomes united with knowledge, emerging from a state of consciousness which is not conditioned by fear and judgement, but accepting of how things are. From here all may be revealed, so that the present can come fully to life.

Nourishing Well-being

Let food be your medicine
and medicine be your food.

HIPPOCRATES

We are nourished by our taste for life. Food, sex and appetites of all sorts provide the ingredients for the feast; it is our responsibility as we mature to turn them into a meal which genuinely fulfils us. Milestones in life such as birthdays, marriages and deaths usually involve eating food especially prepared for the occasion. Eating meals together can strengthen the bonds of relationship; one of the signs of its breakdown is when food is taken separately. Food and sex are intimately linked; lovers with a healthy appetite for eating often have a similar taste for one another.

Nourishing ourselves well involves feeding both our bodies and minds with the best food available in the most agreeable setting. Food that is cooked with care and appreciation, and is arranged beautifully, stimulates the appetite and makes the act of eating all the more satisfactory. Taking time to savour food in a hospitable environment enhances the whole process, so that every time we eat, we eat consciously and celebrate life.

Exercising discrimination in choosing what we need to feed our minds can produce similarly satisfying results. We thrive psychologically when we absorb knowledge that has meaning for us and integrate it so that it becomes part of our being. We need to discover which patterns of thinking cause us harm so that we can find ways to refrain from them and reframe our mental processes, seeking professional help when necessary.

The Four Roles as They Relate to the Solar Plexus Chakra

The digestive system is activated through the solar plexus chakra, releasing the hormone insulin which maintains the blood sugar levels in the body. When the sweetness of life becomes sour it affects our ability to take care of ourselves and to recognize the true value of our own worth. We are fulfilled by what we love and diminished by what we fear. Nourishment can take on many forms, from the food and drink, so essential to the body, to the thoughts which feed the mind and the intentions which gratify the soul. What we eat gives us food for thought; what we drink gives us a thirst for life, which is developed through what we experience in a way that is unique to each of us. This is education in discernment, in finding out what benefits us and what causes harm. Painful experiences which are unresolved can create layers of anxiety which accumulate in the solar plexus, affecting both the external and internal digestive systems. Unsuitable food, full of sugar, salt and saturated fats, cannot be thoroughly digested by the body. Similarly, distressing experiences cannot be processed by the mind until they are recognized and released.

One of the major contributory factors to the holding of tension comes about from roles often established in the family during childhood; such as 'the clever one' who is expected to achieve high academic success, the one who is apportioned much blame, the rebellious one and the family peacemaker. These roles may be maintained subconsciously in adult life. When they cannot be relinquished, either through lack of awareness or resistance to change, they may create a conflict between the past and the present, because they do not relate to current circumstances.

There may be a tendency in those of sanguine disposition to take on the role of interrogator when they are in dialogue with themselves or others. The airy nature

The four roles as they relate to the solar plexus chakra

Element	Humour	Temperament	Nature	Role
Air	Blood	Sanguine	Responsive	Interrogator
Water	Phlegm	Phlegmatic	Sensitive	Victim
Fire	Yellow bile	Choleric	Active	Controller
Earth	Black bile	Melancholic	Receptive	Recluse

can be very forceful in expression and ungrounded ideas may fly in every direction. When this tendency becomes habitual it can generate a relentless velocity which may antagonize or overwhelm others, unwittingly creating conflict. It often needs to find a considerable strength of focus to harness ideas.

The role of interrogator, which the sanguine disposition may assume, can place the listener in a subordinate position so that they feel intimidated and defensive. This questioning nature needs to anchor its ideas by allowing space to listen to responses, internally and externally, so that they can become useful and productive. If this role draws on the element of water to become more sensitive to reactions from others, and to the element of fire to generate warmth it can become well tempered and grounded in the way that it communicates its ideas.

There may be an inclination in those of phlegmatic disposition to take on the role of victim and to seek someone who will solve all their problems. The watery nature may be very self-indulgent, becoming so attached to its difficulties that it cannot see any way out of them. It loses all sense of its own boundaries and it is only through being listened to that they may be re-established, by taking charge of their own feelings. This process may draw on the element of air to clear the mind, fire to warm the heart, and earth to create a sense of security, so that the natural limits can be reformed through being listened to without judgement or unasked-for advice.

There may be a propensity in those of a choleric disposition to take on the role of controller, ordering and influencing situations through the power of energy in them that is inflamed by hidden or revealed anger. The choleric nature may be tempered by elements of water to reduce the flames of impulsive action and earth to provide the place of retreat where anger may subside, allowing more rational thoughts to emerge. Anger may then perform its natural function which is to create a protective shield in times of danger and, drawing on the element of air, inspire the vision for change.

There may be an aptitude in those of a melancholic disposition to distance themselves from others, becoming aloof and unapproachable, even to those whom they hold most dear. The melancholic nature can sink into the ground, creating a hiding place where it may protect itself so that it does not encounter any further difficulties. This sense of isolation is softened by the elements of water, lifted by air and warmed by fire so that it may emerge from the dark into the light when the conditions have become stabilized.

Roles may describe but should never ultimately define us, because they limit our potential for taking on others which are more suited to the moment. Roles allow us to play a part so that we can express ourselves in the moving picture show of events that unfold in our lives. The speech on the seven ages of man in Shakespeare's *As You Like It* declares ' each man in his time plays many parts'; in order to move through all these stages we need to be able to take on different roles so that we do not 'lose the plot' and become disconnected from real meaning in our lives. Trying to assume a position of any kind which is not a conscious, considered response demands a considerable amount of energy which may be better employed elsewhere. We may take on outdated roles many times until we are educated by them in the need to become more flexible and responsive to present requirements. We learn to adapt by learning discernment – physically, psychologically and spiritually. The more we practise it the more we begin to recognize our real worth as human beings, who have not only been given life but also the resources to nurture it throughout every eventuality.

Nourishing well-being through the four roles as they relate to the solar plexus chakra

Manifesting as:	Digesting by:	Manifesting as:	Digesting by:
Air – interrogator		**Fire – controller**	
relentless questions	allowing time for them to be absorbed	becomes overorganized	allowing 'brainstorming'
manipulating conversations	chewing over the main topic	always wanting to take the lead	recognizing others' skills
inflexible attitudes	reflecting them back	interferes with arrangements	respecting choices
unrealistic expectations	assimilating them in the light of the past	urging immediate action	practising reflection
Water – victim		**Earth – recluse**	
seeks to blame	accepting personal responsibilities	prefers solitude to company	becoming observant in company
becomes very dependent	seeking professional help, e.g. psychotherapy	deeply entrenched habits	introducing changes gently
acts very defensively	exploring what causes intolerance	acts very protectively	letting guard down slowly
consumed by sadness	speaking to process it	tendency towards pessimism	eliminating negative experiences safely

The Seven Steps to Emotional Strength

Within the context of the paradigm which is shown in the table 'Energy through Light into Form', on page 14 the seven steps to emotional strength are activated by the nerves, which enable physical and psychological sensations to be experienced and processed through the brain. Emotions can have a powerful impact on the mind, taking precedence over the other faculties of consciousness such as the intellect. Just as physical pain caused by inflammation or obstruction to the nerves can generate the most acute and piercing pain, so psychological suffering can have a similar effect causing a distress that is profoundly debilitating in mind and body. Those who feel emotions deeply and who are unable to express them clearly, or who act them out inappropriately are sometimes referred to as 'nervy' or highly strung. However, when emotions are accepted as an aspect of consciousness, rather than as the whole of it, they can fulfil their function by becoming indicators of issues that need to be addressed, with the support of the other faculties of consciousness. The relationship between the nerves and responses in the seven steps to emotional strength are summarized below.

Cerebral cortex:	give thanks for life itself.
Hypothalamus:	allow time for reflection on a regular basis.
Cervical ganglia medulla:	share feelings with others to develop a greater understanding of how they affect us.
Heart plexus:	look to the whole person before focusing on the partial source of any conflict.
Solar plexus:	examine feelings through reflection rather than reaction.
Sacral plexus:	develop creative skills as an outlet for the expression of feelings.
Coccygeal:	explore the connection between feelings and physical well-being.

Opening up to the meaning of emotional responses requires patience, tolerance, acceptance and education in self-awareness. Emotions are powerful catalysts in the interplay amongst the four elements: they can generate an intensity of feelings which does not dissolve until they have been resolved. This does not happen initially through analysis, which comes under the influence of the brow chakra, but through the solar plexus in the experience of them. Within every feeling there is an underlying cause, which may be repressed or revealed by being acted out subconsciously or through conscious self-examination. Patience draws on the reflective aspect of the element of earth to take on the reclusive role which can be so necessary for self-examination. Tolerance dampens the tendency of the choleric nature towards judgement using a compassion that comes from the sensitivity of the water element. This is applied to the whole person rather than to what is partial in them. Acceptance emerges when the function of a role is seen as transient rather than permanent. This is clarified by the intellectual capacity inspired by the element of air which can examine both rational and irrational modes of behaviour. Education in self-awareness begins with questions that set the whole process in motion, continuing with the willingness to listen to how one feels, developing when a sense of purpose emerges and becoming stabilized through understanding, allowing feelings to play their full part in the expression of consciousness.

The way in which we respond to the feelings of others is a mirror to how we respond to our own. For example, when we are dismissive or critical towards others, we may similarly be denying or judging our own emotions. On the other hand, an open-minded approach accepts emotions as they are, be they habitual or spontaneous. In learning to distinguish between the two, emotions can be put in their rightful place in the development of self-awareness, that process which unmasks our true nature and the roles we adopt in order to uncover it. By taking conscious control of our emotions we can exercise choice in how we feel and can enter into a more authentic relationship with ourselves.

Feelings affect our choices in the food we eat, and our attitude towards eating can have a profound effect on our emotions. In choosing what we eat it is preferable to conform to the body's blood chemistry. Protein foods such as meat, poultry, fish and dairy produce require an acid medium for digestion, whilst carbohydrates in the form of starches and sugars need one which is alkaline. It is helpful to the digestive system to eat meals that are either predominately composed of protein or carbohydrates, rather than being mixed together, so that their nutrients may be fully broken down and assimilated into the bloodstream. Proteins combined with fats draw on insulin in measured amounts, generating energy which is vigorous and enduring, whilst carbohydrates combined with fats create an upsurge of energy, requiring intense amounts of insulin which need to be replenished more quickly to maintain similar effects. When fully utilized, proteins are stimulating and carbo-hydrates relaxing in their relationship with energy. Both need to be selected according to the time of day and what is required to produce essential fuel.

Food combining is of particular help in disorders relating to the digestive and elimina-tion systems, because it enables the nutrients in food to be utilized to their full capacity, so that they can support the process of healing.

Basic Guidelines

- ◆ Do not eat proteins and carbohydrates at the same time.

- ◆ Eat small amounts of proteins and carbohydrates.

- ◆ Eat two to four times as many vegetables as proteins or carbohydrates.

- ◆ Eat fruit between meals.

- ◆ Eat unrefined carbohydrates: bread, cereals, pasta, potatoes, rice.

- ◆ Avoid refined carbohydrates: processed sugars and starches.

- ◆ Avoid all processed fats: hydrogenated fats and oils.

Major food groups

Protein
Eggs
Fish
Meat & poultry
Milk, cheese & yoghurt
Fruits – except bananas, dates and grapes
Pulses
Dry cider & red/white wine

Neutral
Butter & olive oil
Honey
Mayonnaise
Seeds & nuts – except peanuts
Salad & herbs
Vegetables – except potatoes
Gin & whisky

Carbohydrate
Eggs – yolks only
Fats
Milk
Sweet fruits – bananas, dates, figs, grapes, pears, raisins, papaya
Whole grains – barley, buckwheat, millet, oats, rice, wheat
Ale & beer

According to the scientific research carried out during the last 50 years by Dr James D'Adamo and his son Dr Michael D'Adamo, (*Eat Right for your Type* by Peter D'Adamo and Catherine Whitney) our blood groups reflect the roles that we select in the playing out of our lives. The most ancient type, 'O', is the blood of the hunter-gatherer who needs the fire of the choleric temperament with its self-reliant nature to seek foods such as animal flesh, fruits and vegetables for survival. Their digestive systems provided ample amounts of hydrochloric acid for assimilation and to destroy harmful microorganisms.

121

Blood type 'A' evolved as people began to settle and cultivate the land, drawing on the earthy elements of the melancholic temperament, so that they could establish boundaries in which to make their own homes. As their energies were focused in one place there was less meat to eat, so their stomachs began to produce less hydrochloric acid, responding better to vegetables, fruits, grains and fish. There were no cattle as yet to produce milk and its associated dairy products, so there was no adaptation to its ingestion. As land settlements grew and prospered, the increasing population generated the need for expansion and groups seeking new territories became nomadic. These nomads drew on the airy temperament of the flexible nature, which is predominantly peace-loving, seeking not to conquer but to adapt to new domains. This reflected itself in the blood type 'B' which evolved through the adaptation to new and changing conditions by finding a balance between types O and A. Blood type B produced enough hydrochloric acid to digest flesh and fowl as well as grains and dairy produce.

Around a thousand years ago a new blood type, 'AB', emerged, which was a combination of A and B, which developed to meet the changing conditions of the new millennium. The development of this group drew from the elements of water in the charismatic temperament, to delve deep into life with passionate intensity. Their digestive systems adapted to digest most flesh, fish and fowl, as well as grains and dairy produce, but in smaller proportions as they did not produce large amounts of hydrochloric acid in their stomachs. They are natural 'grazers', benefiting from short but regular intakes of small amounts of food to maintain the correct balance in their blood-sugar levels.

Blood-type Characteristics

O	Old	The hunter-gatherer Choleric humor Self-reliant nature
A	Agrarian	The cultivator Air humour Co-operative nature
B	Balance	The nomad Melancholic humour Flexible nature
AB	Adaptor behaviour	The enigma Phlegmatic humour Charismatic nature

Blood carries the life force of both the present and the past. Not only does it transport vital nutrients to every part of the body but also essential memories of what nourishes it, so that it can maintain us to the best of its being.

Since we digest food and feelings through the energy of the solar plexus it is necessary to consider both in terms of nourishing well-being. Just as we need food for our outer strength so we need emotional support for inner robustness. The physical appetite diminishes with states of distress and usually reappears when they are resolved. We feel emotions before we think; they act as searchlights to our inner being. The more we allow ourselves to release our emotions by sharing rather than acting them out, the more we may discover the roles we adopt and the parts we play in life.

Expressive Phrases

Phrases used which relate to our bodies are often a reflection of our state of mind. They may be spoken without much conscious thought but, once heard, can offer a considerable insight into how we are caring for ourselves on a daily basis. Through attunement we can learn from our bodies and find further information about how to relieve any stress that is being held, so that all the parts can be eased into harmony with one another.

The table below on expressive phrases is given as a guideline to the meaning of body parts, but not as a definitive statement. Since our body is in a constant state of flux with the endless interplay between the external and internal environments, the insights that it releases relate to what is happening in the present. Gathering information about it helps to expand our awareness but specific circumstances will always dictate the immediate outcome. Examples of phrases linked to parts of the body are listed below.

Expressive Phrases

Blood	it makes my blood boil	Liver	lily-livered
Head	headstrong	Kidneys	feel it in my water
Skin	itching to do it	Womb	empty nest
Face	can't face it	Testicles	no balls
Hair	hair-brained	Anus	pain in the backside
Eyes	seeing eye-to-eye	Bones	no backbone
Ears	lend an ear	Muscles	muscle in
Nose	being nosey	Joints	being disjointed
Mouth	heart in mouth	Back	can't stand it
Teeth	can't get my teeth into it	Shoulders	carry the burden
Chin	keep my chin up	Arms	keep at arm's length
Neck	pain in the neck	Wrist	tight-fisted
Throat	lump in my throat	Hands	a handful
Chest	weight off my chest	Legs	not a leg to stand on
Heart	heartless	Knees	bowing to the inevitable
Stomach	eaten up inside	Ankles	an ankle biter
Gut	feelings	Feet	put my foot in it

Healing Nutrition

The act of healing absorbs energy in its essential state so that it may be directed to where refuelling is required. This process makes itself known through stomach and intestinal sounds, from both patient and practitioner, showing that activity on a physical level is really taking place. It allows feelings which have been absorbed but not digested to rise to the surface or be fully assimilated so that they may no longer cause obstruction in the energy field. This releases more energy which can be used to develop discernment in both what we need to absorb and discard, and which lies at the heart of all nourishment.

2.8

Accepting Change

Be the change you want to see.

MAHATMA GANDHI

Change is measured in human beings through the growth and development which takes place during their lives. Whilst physical growth is usually achieved by the age of 21, psychological development is a lifetime's work. The processes of change and growth take place most effectively when love is present. It can be inhibited through poor nutrition, an unsupportive environment and traumatic life events such as accidents and bereavements.

The milestones in human growth and development are essentially cyclical in nature. Between the first and last stages there is an enormous range and flexibility of progress; for example, a child facing terminal illness may pass through all the stages in a few months, which might usually happen in a life span of 70 years. An adult in body may be an infant at heart, because the journey to maturity has been halted during childhood. Change activates us, whether it is welcome or not, whereas resistance holds us back, preventing us from developing the characteristics that will support us on our way.

The Four Characters as They Relate to the Sacral Chakra

The sacral chakra determines the four functions of growth, maturation, destruction and renewal. It relates to creativity in all its forms because it contains the urinary organs which regulate the life force through the adrenal glands and the reproductive organs which renew it. It is the urinary system that

The four characters as they relate to the sacral chakra

Element	Humour	Temperament	Nature	Role	Character
Air	Blood	Sanguine	Responsive	Interrogator	Perfectionist
Water	Phlegm	Phlegmatic	Sensitive	Victim	Martyr
Fire	Yellow bile	Choleric	Active	Controller	Intimidator
Earth	Black bile	Melancholic	Receptive	Recluse	Rescuer

allows the blood to be purified, removing toxins to prepare the conditions for the continual cycle of change.

How we respond to change is influenced by the characters that we develop when the roles we have taken on become entrenched. A character is like a seal which stamps our distinctive nature and sets us apart from others. There are characters in literature who are archetypal expressions of the four elements. For example, Gandalf in *The Lord of the Rings* and Ariel in *The Tempest* express the mercurial qualities of the element of air; Viola in *Twelfth Night* and Pierre Bezukov in *War and Peace* express the chameleon-like qualities in the element of water; Scarlett O'Hara in *Gone with the Wind* and D'Artagnan in *The Three Musketeers* are clear expressions of the vigorous quality in the element of fire whilst the eponymous Hamlet and Jane Eyre demonstrate the deep introspective qualities of the element of earth.

The role of the interrogator, for example, may become characterized as that of a perfectionist whose ideals demand order that may be at odds with the modes of everyday life. The energy called upon in seeking to make things perfect is often in conflict with the natural flow of events which reveals the best arrangements in their own times. The sense of frustration that this may engender may cause the headstrong character of the perfectionist to become prone to illnesses affecting the airways and circulatory systems such as asthma, migraines and high blood pressure.

The role of the victim, however, may become characterized in that of a martyr who is defined by the suffering that is experienced to such an extent that it colours every other aspect of life. In this extremely self-involved state a person can become oblivious to the effect it has on others. However, when this condition is met with empathy and compassion the underlying fears may be released and resolved. The lessons learned through this can often be transformative and helpful in supporting others in similar conditions of distress. Left unattended, the state can contribute to such conditions as tension headaches and back and kidney problems.

The role of the controller may become characterized by that of the intimidator, who frightens others into behaviour that denies them freedom of choice. When such control is directed inwards it can constrict energy until it explodes in violent anger or in ferocious self-denial, neither of which recognizes subtle shifts of change. This formidable energy needs to find challenging enterprises to utilize its powers of leadership. When used thoughtfully it may inspire others into effective action without seeking to dominate them. Creative use of such energy can also dissolve the self-destructive anger which, if not addressed, can accumulate, and lay the foundations for future ill health, particularly in inflammatory disorders of the digestive system, such as indigestion, ulcers and diverticulitis.

The role of the recluse may become characterized as that of a rescuer, who seeks to save others with heroic deeds. These acts can still preserve the distance which is so vital to those who are reclusive by nature because they are grand gestures which do not necessarily impinge on the smaller details of life. Having made the grand gesture they are gone to save another soul, loving the idea of mankind in general, but wary of intimacy in particular. This energy may become earthed by being nurtured through gentle, regular exposure to social interaction, allowing the time and space for practical involvement and reflective observation, so that relationships once kept at bay eventually become welcomed and accepted. Such engagement reduces the predisposition towards states of depression which can be generated through isolation.

We may adopt many characters in our lives to accommodate changing times. It is a part of our life pattern to question and seek order, to share our pleasures and difficulties, to fight for what we believe in and to withdraw from time to time. Problems arise when we become caricatures of ourselves, exaggerated versions of what were once authentic responses but which are no longer viable. It is only through facing ourselves as we really are that we can look into the mirror of our own being. The writer Colette said, 'look a long time at what pleases you and longer still at what pains you'. If we are willing to evaluate ourselves we open up to a process of continuous personal discovery which does not seek self-aggrandizement, but turns towards self-awareness, drawing on all the innate resources that are always available for change, to bring about the best arrangement for well-being.

Accepting change through the four characters as they relate to the sacral chakra

Manifesting as:	Regulating by:	Manifesting as:	Regulating by:
Air – perfectionist		**Fire – intimidator**	
fixed ideals	studying philosophical and spiritual texts	natural leader	learning management skills
demands proof	analysing scientific research	strong opinions	allowing others to express theirs
high achiever	seeking satisfaction in practical skills	prefers to speak rather than listen	learning how to listen
never fulfilled	practising meditation and relaxation	strong physical energy	exercising regularly
Water – martyr		**Earth – rescuer**	
defined by suffering	seeking humour to lighten mood	romantic ideals	learning about relationships
frightened of change	sharing fears	distaste for emotions	studying emotional intelligence
drawn to suffering of others	working in healthcare	unapproachable	making contact with someone every day
uses emotional blackmail	studying assertiveness skills	very methodical	acting spontaneously

The Seven Ages of Humankind

Within the context of the paradigm which is shown in the table 'Energy through Light into Form', on page 14 the seven ages of humankind are set in motion by the hormones that relate to each body process. Whilst the seven stages of humankind adapt and evolve according to life experience, their potential within every being is not limited by time but only by the inability to be receptive to what is possible and to allow changes to come about that can increase understanding in the light of new experiences.

The changes that demarcate the seven ages of humankind evolve through an organic process of growth, maturation, destruction and renewal prior to embarking on the next stage of development. This process is reflected in both the macrocosm and the microcosm; through the seasons of spring, summer, autumn and winter in the exterior, and in the interior composition of every cell in the body. If all the phases are not completed, they leave traces behind which affect the subsequent levels, diminishing their ability to reach their full potential. Every age sows the seeds for spiritual awareness, which directs the emotional, intellectual and physical intelligences towards self-discovery. In the period of growth there is the necessity for self-preservation which is essential to develop the body and mind. In maturation there is the need for self-endurance, so necessary at times for protection against the trials and tribulations of living. Through destruction there is the grief of loss and the sense of self-desolation that it may engender, which is none the less inevitable because it has to make way for the new, the reality of every instant of creation that is never the same as the one preceding it.

The formulation of character can be held back when there is a delay or even a halt in this process through physical, psychological or spiritual trauma. The perfectionist may be trapped by the fear of failure; the martyr by the longing to be understood. The intimidator may be in desperate need of self-control and the rescuer unable to find a way to be rescued. Only when these characteristics are recognized by those subject to them can there be insight as to how they came about. In this way choice is opened up, which is the key to the gate that encloses the imprisoned self.

According to the understanding that we have existence before conception and after death, our appearance in this realm enables each of us to realize our full potential through the unique configuration of our body, mind and soul. The self

The hormones as they relate to the seven ages of man

Hormone	Standing	Action
Articular e.g. adrenaline; cortisone	Age of experience	Introducing the senses of the body
Regulatory e.g. oestrogen; progesterone; testosterone	Age of reason	Developing the faculties of the mind
Digestive e.g. insulin; glycogen	Age of assimilation	Applying discernment gained from practical experiences in everyday life
Circulatory e.g. thymosin	Age of acceptance	Coming to acknowledge oneself in both weaknesses and strengths
Respiratory e.g. thyroxine	Age of inspiration	Following the courage of one's convictions
Hypothalmic e.g. pituitrin	Age of balance	Seeking harmony within oneself in body, mind and soul
Cerebral e.g. melatonin	Age of awareness	Becoming conscious of oneself

is fully established in all of its possibilities prior to birth, in a similar way to the potential for a building, which becomes established by virtue of the architect's plans. This does not, however, impose predestination or negate free will. Living our life is the bringing out of that potential through freedom of choice and making it real in this world, in all its scope and detail.

The self is at once fully established before time and yet expresses itself both generally and specifically in time in the seven ages of humankind. There are recognizable phases in humankind, beginning with a developing awareness of one's own self as an individual, distinct from others, which occurs in early childhood, followed by the need to establish relationships which encourage self-respect. If these flourish they support the self in finding its value and learning how to protect it from harm. From the security of self-acceptance there arises the courage to speak from the heart, in the knowledge that it is only through the truth that any real sense of self-awareness can continue to manifest.

The self perpetuates its journey from awareness to knowledge through the continuous cycle of change which never ends in its journey through life. Resistance to development may reveal itself, for example, in postnatal depression in both women and men, which may have its roots in experiences of inadequate parenting when in childhood; similarly, the reason for an inability to support a partner in their role as new mother or father may be tracked back through childhood memories of rejection or abandonment. The movement of energy through the self is summarized below.

Self-awareness: through its mindfulness of the physical body in its earthly surroundings.

Self-respect: through its capacity to create productive relationships with others and with oneself.

Self-worth: through its ability to discriminate between what is harmful or beneficial for oneself and others.

Self-acceptance: through its capacity for courage in the face of adversity, when it is open to life rather than closed off from it.

Self-expression: through its power to communicate the experience of love by speaking from the heart.

Self-responsibility: through its ability to respond to the needs of the self.

Self-consciousness: through its potential to be aware of oneself as a whole person.

When adults demonstrate child-like behaviour which is damaging both to themselves and others, it is helpful for them to explore the reasons for their actions. One method of exploration is to travel back in time to childhood, to work with 'the inner child' and to see what memories emerge, which may help us to understand our current behaviour. In this setting we become our own parent, giving ourselves the care that only we can provide. The parent that we have become is the one that is the most effective for us because it is born out of love and compassion; love for ourselves beyond condition and compassion that allows it to come wholly into being.

Reflection on the Needs of your Inner Child

- Sit quietly.
- Take a few deep breaths.
- Allow yourself to descend into a deeper level of consciousness.
- Ask for permission to meet your inner child.
- Greet yourself as a child.
- Ask your inner child what age he or she is.
- Sit with your child and allow memories to emerge.
- Witness them together.
- Hold your child and enfold him or her with loving thoughts.
- Stay with your inner child until he or she is ready to leave.
- Come back into familiar consciousness.
- Give thanks for your experience.
- Check that you are grounded.
- Move forward!

Another method of exploration is to recall significant dreams which stay fresh in the mind and ask what meaning is contained within them. Dreams generally emerge from our subconscious which works only with images. They may present as a jumble of pictures, as a sequence of events or even as insights into the future. An image is like a photograph which has been fully developed; it is complete in itself. It cannot be adjusted and can therefore represent itself clearly. Just as photographs can be very revealing so can dreams, for they show to us what is happening in the deeper levels of our minds. If we want to understand what is within ourselves we need to use all the faculties of consciousness, which includes our dreams, so that we can explore their meaning through the information which is not always accessible to the conscious mind.

Practical Guidelines for Dream Analysis

- ◆ Keep a dream diary.
- ◆ Keep writing paper and a pencil by the bedside.
- ◆ Record your dreams as soon as you wake up.
- ◆ Record any words that you hear during your sleep or as you awaken.
- ◆ Allow your dreams to inform you of their meaning by asking them to reveal their underlying message.
- ◆ Seek professional help if you feel it is necessary.
- ◆ Do not accept the interpretation of your dream by another person unless it meets with acceptance in you.

When we recognize the need for change it is a sign of strength to seek help. Whether we turn to family, friends or professional therapists for support, we need to feel safe with the person whose help we seek; if there are any persistent doubts it is better to go elsewhere. Feelings serve our senses; they transport physical impressions into the light of the mind so that it can interpret them, and illuminate the way that guides us towards well-being.

All growth may be inhibited by self-indulgence, when boundaries are not sufficiently established to provide the right setting to nourish it. Equally, maturation may not take place fully if self-esteem becomes replaced by self-satisfaction and self-promotion rather than a willingness to evaluate oneself honestly on a regular basis. Destruction produces debris which needs processing so that it can be removed. Debris which is not removed becomes toxic; if the body or the mind holds on to toxic matter there can be no movement and change is prevented.

Without change there can be no renewal, which is essential for the completion of this cycle and the beginning of the next one. Renewal occurs most effectively when the self is in its centre, balanced and ready for the changes that lie ahead.

Expressive Muscles

Information about how the body feels can be discovered by applying pressure on the muscles, as in the practice of kinesiology. Every muscle group is supplied with energy through the meridians, which have both a physical and a psychological effect on the related body organs. For example, the muscles in the arm receive their energy through the fire and metal meridians; the former is associated with enthusiasm for living and the latter with an underlying sense of loss or grief. When applying kinesiology in this way the arm is held out to the side of the body at shoulder level, and then pressed downwards by another person, firmly but without exerting undue strength. If the muscles in the arm remain strong under pressure they indicate the quality of energy which is received through the first and second fire meridians, namely the heart and small intestine, and the triple heater and heart protector. The visible strength in the muscles reflects their inner ability to respond with the expansive energy of fire to what is being tested. If the arm moves downwards when pressed it reflects the influence of the meridians of the lung and large intestine which are associated with all the functions of elimination, both in body and mind, and thus indicate a letting-go or a resistance in response to what is being tested. This technique can be used for making choices through every level of energy in:

spiritual education:	taking courses in personal development, philosophical programmes or religious studies.
recalling memories:	seeking help through counselling, behavioural or psychotherapies or psychiatric support.
asking questions:	making decisions about work conditions, travel plans or social activities.
affirming choices:	declaring intentions about nutrition, lifestyle or environment.
checking reactions:	investigating responses to eating programmes, living arrangements or cultural influences.

confirming medication:	testing the suitability of vitamins and mineral supplements, herbal and homeopathic remedies or allopathic medication.
organizing exercise:	planning suitable regimes for body toning and shaping, physical sports or subtle energy practices.

This process requires a willing participant to conduct the investigation, which may proceed as follows:

◆ Bring an issue to mind which needs clarification.

◆ If testing for allergic reaction to food or drink take hold of the specific item, for example: bread, milk or wine.

◆ Extend the arm sideways.

◆ Allow the participant to exert a gentle but firm downwards pressure on the forearm.

◆ Resist the pressure being exerted on it without letting the arm become rigid.

◆ Observe the reaction in the arm.

◆ If the arm remains in position there is sufficient energy to support the situation, such as in the body's ability to digest a particular food or drink.

◆ If the arm falls there is insufficient energy to maintain it and the food or drink concerned should be avoided.

There can be no movement without muscles. They work in pairs, expanding and contracting throughout the body so that it is in a perpetual state of flux. Many of these movements take place at a subconscious level through the autonomic system. However, the more conscious we become of the continuum of energy, which manifests through the mind into every facet of the body – in this instance through the muscles – the greater the involvement we can bring by making choices which enhance rather than diminish their ability to support us to the best of their being.

Healing Change

The act of healing facilitates change. It provides a source of support so that patients can access their own inner strength and external resources, which are necessary to make change happen. The role of the practitioner is not to influence the changes that need to take place but to help maintain the focus so that the patient can make the best choice possible to set them in motion. This offers a renewed sense of purpose to follow through what has been received during the treatment and for the decisions to be integrated into the patient's life.

2.9

Exercising Energy

Man has no Body distinct from his Soul.

WILLIAM BLAKE, *THE MARRIAGE OF HEAVEN AND HELL*

One of the meanings of the word 'exercise' is 'to make use of'. Within the context of healthcare for the whole person, exercise can be seen as making use of all the bioenergetic systems, from the most dense, which are the body organs, to the most subtle, the meridians, chakras and the aura.

The human body is in a constant state of movement; it is a workhouse of activity in which growth, maturation, destruction and renewal takes place, without ceasing, from conception until death. It may take as long as seven years or as short a time as nine months for whole systems, apart from the central nervous system, to be renewed; for example, liver cells are replaced every 6 weeks, skin cells every 28 days and the intestinal tract cells every 36 hours. There is a natural rhythm within the systems of the body which consists of expansion, contraction and pause, as exemplified in the action of the heart and lungs, allowing movement to take place within a balance of action and stillness. The healthy human heart is said to require 12 hours' work and 12 hours' rest, so that in a 24-hour cycle there should be 8 hours of sleep to support 8 hours of work and 4 hours of relaxation. Such a balance is at the heart of all effective exercise; too much depletes the immune system and damages the physical organs, too little slows down the flow of energy and the body's metabolic rate.

The need for exercise is always balanced by the requirement for rest. During the four hours of relaxation it is highly beneficial to adopt the semi-supine position recommended by the Alexander technique for 20 minutes, once or twice a day. This position involves lying on the floor with the head resting on a book. The position should be comfortable with no undue pressure being exerted on the head or the neck. The knees are bent, legs hip-width apart and hands resting on the ribs. This position allows the vertebrae to receive their full quota of blood, enabling the peripheral nerves, which transmit sensations from the spinal cord into the organs of the body, to function to their greatest ability. It aligns the head, neck and body so that the energy which fuels them may move fully and freely throughout the entire length and breadth of the physical form.

Further balance between exercise and rest can be helped through developing creative skills. These can also be complemented by periods of contemplation. The active imagination often lies buried unless used consciously, for example by those who use creativity in their work. Contemplation and meditation may free the imagination to surface from the depths of consciousness. The more work there is to complete, the greater the benefit of meditation, which settles the senses and calms the mind, so that they can be replenished in a peaceful setting. The harder one drives oneself the more urgent it becomes to stand back in reflection, to assess what really matters in life.

The Four Selves in the Base Chakra

The self is our personal organizer, without which we have no identity; it is the actor within us, which can take on many parts. Its ability to cast itself in the right part at the right time is influenced by what it has inherited from ancestral memory and from its own experiences in this world. The presence of unresolved pain causes energy to become blocked and so inhibits full self-expression. When this becomes visible it can be released, allowing the self to draw more freely on all its resources in body, mind and soul, so that it can make full use of them.

The four selves in the base chakra

Element	Humour	Temperament	Nature	Role	Character	Self
Air	Blood	Sanguine	Responsive	Interrogator	Perfectionist	Philosopher
Water	Phlegm	Phlegmatic	Sensitive	Victim	Martyr	Visionary
Fire	Yellow bile	Choleric	Active	Controller	Intimidator	Pioneer
Earth	Black bile	Melancholic	Receptive	Recluse	Rescuer	Peacemaker

This is the whole self that is integrated and is able to maintain a balance between its external and internal environment. It is ever present, waiting to be discovered in the depth of every being – ready to make itself known through every life experience.

The character that is driven by air through the power of the intellect to formulate abstract ideals of perfection can be transposed into the self that is a philosopher, whose understanding becomes imbued with a love of wisdom. When theories become actualized within this context they may find their proper place in the scheme of events because they have taken into account the vagaries as well as the recognized patterns of the human condition.

The character under the influence of water, who may often take on the role of victim, may be transformed from the self of a martyr to that of a visionary whose own experience of difficulty and pain enables them not only to empathize with others but to be of practical help to them because they have the emotional intelligence and compassion that comes from a depth of understanding.

The character in whom fire is prevalent, and who can be ablaze with such fervour that it may predominate over the other natures, can be transformed into the self of a pioneer, when enthusiasm is tempered with patience. This energy, which is so well suited to innovatory enterprises, thrives on a structured support which keeps the fire burning but prevents it from getting out of control.

The character under the dominion of earth, who seeks the security of isolation, may be transmuted into the self of a peacemaker because their reflective observations can provide insight into the different temperaments and natures, how they interact with one another and how to bring them into accord with one another.

The transmutation of energy through one appearance into another is an alchemical process involving the nature of elements, humours and temperaments as they devolve into the qualities of roles, characteristics and selfhood. It follows a natural order, which may be witnessed everywhere in life, in the anatomy and physiology of the body and in the patterns and programmes of the mind. Within this order there is a place for both science and art, in the known of what can be measured and in the unknown of what appears to challenge previous definitions and to seek new frontiers of further understanding, which validate both intuition and reason. This is energy at its most dynamic, creative and free-flowing – exercising consciousness so that it may express intelligence in the light of every form.

Exercising energy through the four selves as they relate to the base chakra

Manifesting as:	Moving by:	Manifesting as:	Moving by:
Air – philosopher		**Fire – pioneer**	
seeking explanations	gathering them into an integrated perspective	seeking adventures	travelling regularly
		courageousness in danger	learning survival skills
enjoying mind games	developing left-brain skill by activities such as crosswords, card and board games	leading others	developing management skills
devouring theoretical considerations	observing practical outcomes	preferring action to rest	arranging one restful activity a day
overemphasizing intellectual skills	becoming grounded in sport, dance, martial arts and domestic skills		
Water – visionary		**Earth – peacemaker**	
seeking emotional intelligence	studying positive mental-health practices	seeking tranquillity	practising meditation regularly
developing social contacts	cultivating an active social life	practising negotiation	learning listening and assertiveness skills
thriving in group settings	developing support group and voluntary aid programmes	detachment from conflict	studying history and politics
drawn to spiritual education	practising meditation, attending courses, going into retreat	unobtrusiveness	developing self-confidence in company

The Seven Ways to be Grounded

Within the context of the paradigm which is shown in the table 'Energy through Light into Form', on page 14, the seven ways to be grounded can be found in all seven processes of the body. Being open in mind, alert in readiness to adapt, receptive to inspiration, centred in the heart, prepared to be nourished, willing to change when necessary, and being focused through all the senses, can all be reflected and accessed when the physical body is poised in stillness and yet ready for action. Within this state of being the body is able to do what is required with ease, because it can access energy from the other six levels and utilize it to its maximum potential.

The grounding practice related to each body process

Process	Grounding practice
Sensation	Experiencing life without resistance so that the senses can be fully explored.
Adaptation	Being willing to adjust to changing circumstances.
Respiration	Keeping the lines of communication open, whatever the circumstances.
Circulation	Disengaging from conflict and asking for compassion to move from disease to ease.
Digestion	Guarding oneself against anxiety by not dwelling on the past or planning the future but by giving time to the present.
Regulation	Protecting oneself by not getting over involved in other people's lives.
Articulation	Removing oneself from places that feel unsafe in any way.

We exercise ourselves most completely through our bodies which keep us centered. When we reflect on our bodies we come to know their tendencies, their likes and dislikes, their requirements and how to take the best care of them. Our individual selves require a vehicle for expression and there is none better crafted to suit this purpose than the living form, which can reveal itself through every aspect of its anatomy and physiology. The shape of the head, the colour and composition of the eyes, the state of the tongue, the condition of the nails; all the moving parts display their condition of health.

If the mind is ahead of the body, as may be seen in the character of the perfectionist, it is difficult to become centered within the physical form and hear the information that is coming from it. When the mind is dampened by excessive sadness, for example in feelings of martyrdom or of being ill used, it can become disassociated from the body, exhibiting symptoms such as loss of appetite and lack of interest in anything other than its own self-concern. Alternatively, if the mind is on fire with self-righteousness, as characterized by the controller, which is determined to assert and impose its beliefs at whatever cost, it pays scant regard to the more subtle processes of negotiation and compromise. When the mind is darkened by doubts and lack of confidence a reclusive state prevails; it seeks a place to hide and protect itself, until it finds the ability to emerge into the light of day and face the outer world. This seclusion can be actual and physical or metaphorical and psychological, in the sense of taking refuge in a set of hardened beliefs or opinions which the person is reluctant to relinquish or change.

Our minds reflect the colourings of the characters we are drawn to, but in themselves are essentially colourless, so that they may adapt to the shifting patterns of light that are generated by our thoughts. At the heart of every being is the real self, which in religious and spiritual traditions is described as the place where the human is made in the image of the Divine. This is the self that brings us fully to life, so that what we experience is the whole measure of ourselves. It requires a responsive mind, a sensitive soul, an active body and a self which is receptive to all that it encounters, whatever its temperament or nature. It needs to make use of all the resources at its disposal, which are found in the constitution of the body in infinite supply. This is made possible when the body is brought into alignment with the soul through the light of the mind, so that it can discriminate what is necessary for its well-being and further development.

When the body becomes grounded in its self, it becomes stabilized in its own environment. It can then protect itself properly, because its defence systems, such as the immune services and adrenalin supplies, can be released quickly and effectively as its energy is not being dissipated elsewhere. Without being able to defend ourselves we cannot help to protect others, such as children, in a way that is most suited to their needs or requirements. When, for example, there is an airy dismissal of problems, they are not really blown away; equally, a misplaced flood of empathy can swamp them. Unsolicited attempts to manage other people's problems can be overwhelming and leave them feeling depleted and depressed; excessive sympathy can also be misplaced, engulfing details so that they become obscured.

It becomes more difficult to protect oneself and others when there is an excessive predominance of one element over another. Protection can be highly effective when the elements are in balance with one another, preventing the energy field from becoming damaged by both external and internal sources of danger. Protection is a fundamental need in all of us, from conception until death, so that we are guarded as much as possible against danger in all its forms, both from others and indeed from ourselves. When energy becomes imploded through pathological conditions it can turn inward and become self-destructive, whether through psychological problems resulting in bodily self-harm at one extreme, or through failures in the immune system at the other, which lead to illnesses of the autoimmune system.

Danger is an innate part of life and the reaction to danger is a necessary and instinctive response to anything that poses a threat to the organism. The more

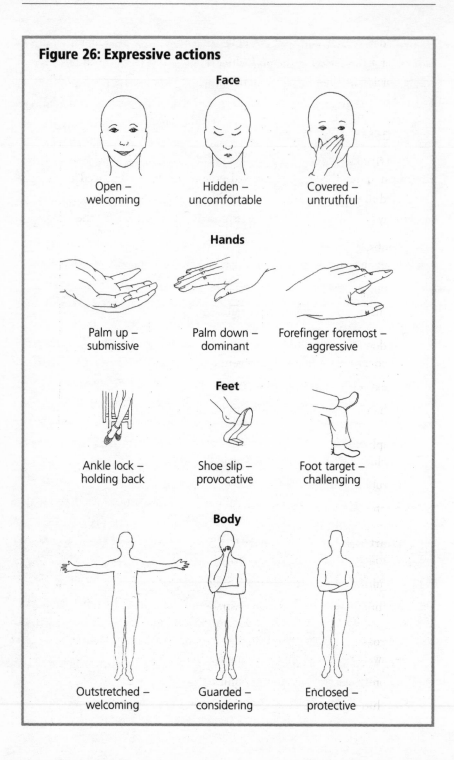

Figure 26: Expressive actions

Face

Open –
welcoming

Hidden –
uncomfortable

Covered –
untruthful

Hands

Palm up –
submissive

Palm down –
dominant

Forefinger foremost –
aggressive

Feet

Ankle lock –
holding back

Shoe slip –
provocative

Foot target –
challenging

Body

Outstretched –
welcoming

Guarded –
considering

Enclosed –
protective

grounded a person is, the more able they are to respond appropriately to whatever arises, meeting the difficulties and challenges of life and recovering more quickly from adverse situations.

Expressive Actions

Actions speak louder than words. We express ourselves through our body at a speed far faster than that of verbal communication. We need to be fully grounded in the present to observe and be educated by body language. Seven areas may be observed to help understand the meaning behind the actions.

Limbs:
- unable to stand still: wanting to get away.
- one leg in front of the other: feeling guarded.
- sitting on the edge of the chair: eager to escape.

Abdomen:
- covering it: protecting the genitals.
- exposing it: to express sexuality.
- hands directed downwards: indicating conflict.

Diaphragm:
- clutching it: to hold in any pain.
- rubbing it: to show pleasure.
- protecting it: to hide feelings.

Heart:
- touching it: to convey sincerity.
- mirroring gestures: to reflect closeness.
- thumbs up over it: to demonstrate superiority.

Throat:
- swallowing frequently: feeling nervous.
- breathing quickly: feeling panicky.
- chin up: feeling defiant.

Brow:

- covering the eyes: to hide the truth.

- blinking regularly: to disconnect from seeing.

- looking into the eyes: radiating attraction.

Head:

- covering it: to control thoughts.

- rubbing it: to clear the mind.

- patting it: to convey patronage.

Our actions express our truth. We may learn to moderate and even control some of our responses for sustained periods of time, but they will only be held in abeyance, not deleted from the body's memory. The language of the body is extremely powerful in its impact and may reveal what words cannot or dare not say. It influences us with a presence which cannot be dispelled; it calls out to be heard and understood, so that it can fulfil its purpose.

Healing Exercise

The act of healing can replenish energy when we have either overexerted or injured ourselves during, for example, excessive exercise programmes. It can also activate energy when it has been underused, such as during periods of depression, when there may be no impetus for movement of any kind. Healing re-establishes the natural order of flow from the interior to the exterior, so that energy may follow the paths designated for it without any obstructions. This invites us to come back into harmony with ourselves, so that we may gain a more realistic perspective about when we need to exercise and how to balance it with rest.

Health for the Whole Person

The health of the whole person is not defined by illness or misfortune but by the responses they evoke. When they are accepted as part of life, they find their place in the scheme of things; if they become the whole matter they overwhelm everything else and leave no room for reflection and healing. How we respond is reflected in the composition of our constitutions, and how we react to them.

When the element of air predominates in a person it can create a web to trap unrealistic expectations of recovery which may not match the reality of what is actually happening. If the element of water is uppermost it may generate a sense of persecution from the feeling of the unfairness of suffering. When the element of fire is the guiding force it can produce a warrior-like response with over-optimism and a fervent determination to battle against all odds and defeat the enemy of sickness. If the element of earth asserts itself excessively over the other three it can cause a person to retreat into a state of deeply entrenched pessimism. When there is an imbalance between the elements of earth and fire, conditions such as migraines may arise, when the enthusiasm of the fiery temperament is suppressed by the stoical nature of earth in whatever condition it finds itself. If there is an imbalance between fire and air, conditions such as asthma may appear, when the heat of the fire burns up the air, depleting the energy of the breath. An imbalance between the elements of air and water can lead to depressive states of mind, because the lightness of air, which invites inspiration, is flooded with feelings of unresolved grief. The unequal combination of the elements of water and earth can lead to spinal problems such as aching in the neck, shoulder and back. Water is associated with fear, and air with stability. When they are out of balance with one another the structures of the body can feel threatened through an accumulated sense of danger, real or illusory.

When the elements of nature are able to resolve these conflicts by finding the way to co-operate with one another, states of distress and illness may be transformed into the status of well-being. The whole person draws on all of them as they are required, for physical, psychological and spiritual energy, as they evolve from elemental to substantial being, as witnessed here on earth.

Section 3

HEALING

3.1

Co-ordinating Health with Healing

Health is a condition in which body, mind and soul work in harmony with one another. In a number of philosophies the human being stands between heaven and earth, moving between them, uniting the two and reflecting both. Real health is a state of being – both elevated, representing heaven, and grounded, representing earth – in which energy circulates from the high to the low, drawing on both to support the life system in all its complexity. In the movement of this energy there is the drawing in of breath, inspiration which relates to elevation, and the absorption of it in the physical form which relates to the actuality of earth.

Although the physical body appears to be solid and fixed, its composition in reality is dynamic. This is designed to bring about a state of health that is flexible, so that it can adapt to the changing conditions within the body itself and in the surrounding environment. It is the resistance to such adaptation, whether reflected through the body or the mind, that interrupts the full flow of energy and causes illness. Within the consciousness of energy there is an innate intelligence which guides and informs it through every breath, in every cell in the body, along the meridians, within the chakras and beyond form into the aura. All seven levels of energy express this intelligence in which the organism has an inherent ability to heal itself.

Negative patterns of thinking which are either inherited through past generations, accumulated by life experience or exercised in the present, can affect this ability for healing. They can diminish the powers of the physical body, corrupting the creative processes of the mind and clouding the receptivity of the soul. Patterns of thinking which appear to be positive but actually cover up the truth of a situation with the pretence that all is well when it is not, can have a similar effect, creating an illusion of well-being which is not valid.

The path to real health goes beyond both negative and positive states of mind, seeking to be conscious of every state which arises, and identifying it without reacting to it. Such conscious thought brings us into the present with an open mind and a receptive soul. It grounds the physical body and the mind in the moment. This is the consciousness of healing, which is open to all possibilities in its potential to ease the body, calm the mind and bring insights from the soul. Healing consciousness is directed by thought – if a request is made for healing, the energy will respond to it and healing begins to take place. In the act of healing it is purity of thought that opens up the healing consciousness to its full potential. Here purity of thought is a request made completely without conditions or expectations of any kind; it is like a blank page waiting for impressions to be inscribed upon it. It emerges through the attunement of the senses of the body and the faculties of the mind gathered in complete receptivity. In this state the healing process is free to take place, leading to the unblocking and rebalancing of energy wherever it is required.

This can be a complex process, working through layers of life experiences that have caused imbalances in the energy field and may not produce immediate relief. Indeed, there may be healing crises, in which the signs and symptoms of previous disorders reappear, causing some difficulties before they are realized and released. The act of healing instigates a natural series of changes that are guided by the unique nature of every being so that it can be both inspired by and educated through whatever it has experienced in life.

Learning about Healing

What has happened will happen again,
and what has been done will be done again;
and there is nothing new under the sun.
Is there anything of which one can say:
'Look, this is new?'

No, it has already existed, long ago
before our time.
The men of old are not remembered, and
those who follow will not be remembered
by those who follow them.

ECCLESIASTES 1:9–11

Healing is as natural as breathing. It is ongoing, whether or not we are aware of it. It may need assistance in the form of medicine or surgery, or support through massage or manipulation, but it works through the mind into the body, to adjust self-destructive patterns of thinking, to seal wounds, to destroy infections, to repair damaged cells and to compensate for structural injuries to the best of its ability.

The energy that is essential for healing may be requested through the power of thought and activated according to the existing conditions within the energy field. This process is one of attunement to the consciousness of the universal healing energy, and is the most ancient and enduring form of healthcare. It happens subconsciously through all sympathetic responses when we identify with another person's distress or illness and reach out to them, when there is real listening or in the reassurance of physical contact. It happens consciously when there is full agreement and co-operation with the practitioner, the patient and the healing energies that come into being.

When healing becomes a conscious act, it needs to be practised with great care and purified intention. One of the first things that a healing practitioner needs to guard against is the idea of 'ability'. The ego can be very subtle in the ways that it tries to appropriate actions and place the practitioner at the centre of the treatment as someone who can 'help' the patient to get better. This is the natural tendency of the ego left to its own devices and we need to be mindful of it so that it can be corrected through self-awareness.

A practitioner should, secondly, guard against the possibility of developing a codependent relationship in which the patient attempts to place the practitioner in a position of influence and the practitioner allows it. This can create an unhealthy situation in which the patient can become dependent on the practitioner, abnegating their freedom of choice and also seeking to involve the practitioner in other areas of their life. There can be an uneasy relationship between those who may be seen to hold power by those who feel beholden to them. This should be addressed through encouraging personal responsibility in the healing context whenever the question of making choices arises. In the past there was often suspicion of healing practitioners who, at various times, were accused of having supernatural powers and abilities to harm as well as those to heal. This is still the case in some societies today. In the not too recent past, accusations of witchcraft led to banishment, imprisonment and even death.

Gradually, over a period of time, the focus in healing moved from the more subtle influences of the meridians and chakras to the anatomy and physiology of the body, which could be understood through its structural components, with little or no reference to the psyche and its processes.

A unifying perspective began to emerge during the 20th century with the theories of relativity, quantum phenomena, chaos and holograms. Fundamental to this work is the understanding that energy comes from a universal source; that it recreates itself; that its behaviour cannot be predicted; and that every cell contains the information of the whole being as in a hologram. This latter principle is reflected in the etheric level of energy that holds the template for every life form, which in itself is made evident in the DNA in every cell of the body, each containing the complete code for recreating life.

These modern expressions of the nature of energy are in accord with the ancient traditions of the chakras, which came through the yogis in India, and the meridians that were annotated by the Taoists in China. They are also consistent with the early Greek physicians – with 'the healing power of nature', as described by Hippocrates, and the integrated perspective of Galen whose diagnostic skills in pulse-taking, for example, reflect that of an acupuncturist combined with those of a physician.

Our understanding of energy and how it affects our health is enriched by the traditions of the past and enhanced by continuing discoveries. We now have access to a formidable amount of information and require an education in healing and healthcare to make the best use of it. Education is an ongoing process and has to be flexible to meet the needs of the time, allowing the form and content of particular programmes or courses to change if necessary. Enduring knowledge is timeless and transcends the passing ages, yet, by absorbing what is relevant from the past and being receptive to what is pertinent in the present, we can look to the future with a broader and deeper frame of reference.

It is a barrier to understanding to think that at a certain point we now 'know' all that we need to know. If we do this, we cut off the possibility of further growth and development. Education at this point does not necessarily involve more training, although this may help, but rather it is a state of mind that allows us to be educated by the work itself. If we are prepared to follow this we can be guided to deeper and more subtle levels of perception, which can only benefit both ourselves and the patients whom we treat.

Education in healing involves:

- learning about the physical and subtle natures of bodies and how to look after them;
- developing co-operative working relationships with other practitioners;
- acquiring skills which increase emotional intelligence;
- finding a balance between work and rest;
- practising conversation skills;
- exploring the psychology of the mind; and
- cultivating a sense of spiritual awareness.

A working knowledge of the structures, functions and subtle energies of the body can offer greater insight to an education in healing. Although study of the details involved is helpful, it is greatly enhanced through the practice of work experience in a professional or voluntary setting such as a hospital or residential home. It is also complemented by first-aid skills and an awareness of potential risks and how to prevent them. A patient can be affected most powerfully through the act of healing and it is important that the practitioner can both understand and respond to any physical or psychological reactions to the work that is taking place.

An education in healing also benefits from learning how to work with others. Developing creative relationships allows students to learn from other practitioners and from each other, so that there is always a sense of exploration within all the subject matter.

Developing emotional intelligence is an important part of training in healing, since so many physical, psychological and spiritual health problems have their roots in unresolved emotional tensions, which cause energy to stagnate in the part of the body where they were first experienced. The more we learn about our own emotional responses, the more we can empathize and support others. All feelings are a driving force for understanding the truth of a particular situation; they can direct us to a far greater awareness when we allow ourselves to be educated through them by opening up to their underlying meanings.

It is also important for all practitioners of healing to learn how to look after themselves before giving their time and attention to others. A balance is required which is helped through developing the practice of the regular self-appraisal that comes from reviewing one's life experiences. It is our responsibility to encourage and develop this self-awareness so that we are better prepared to be of service to the work of healing.

It is beneficial for all practitioners of healing to develop their communication skills in both speaking and listening, so that they can establish a meaningful connection with their patients. There is nothing more helpful than being heard and acknowledged; real listening releases blocked energy, allowing both patient and practitioner to explore the full dimensions of the matter being discussed. They act as mirrors to one another during this time, reflecting their own experiences and understanding through the content of the conversation.

Education in healing also requires study of the functions of the mind and how the power of thought can affect them. Without being able to recognize destructive patterns of thinking, there is no way to change them. They run on unchecked, causing the mind to lose the ability to think constructively. Acute and chronic mental health problems are usually beyond the remit of the healing practitioner, because they require specialist psychiatric care. Treatment should only be given with the permission of the medical staff concerned. Healing work can supplement such medical care by engaging the patient at a deeper level of consciousness, encouraging a profound sense of relaxation and relief, giving some respite from mental turmoil.

There are many situations, however, that do not require psychiatric attention but do benefit from the recognition of these acute and chronic patterns of destructive thinking. When they are recognized they can be reframed with the help of skilled guidance so that the patient can gain a more balanced perspective.

Developing skills to support this process will enable practitioners to complement the work of other professionals, offering healthcare that is wholly integrated in both body and mind.

Education in healing requires a spiritual perspective which both expands the mind and grounds the body, inspired by the natural receptivity of the soul. The education of the shaman, for example, was composed traditionally of 90 per cent spiritual practices and 10 per cent practical work. This emphasizes the necessity for the development of spiritual intelligence, without which fundamental life skills may have no purpose or substantial effect. It encourages the practitioner to explore the connection between spirituality and the practice of healing, so that the reality of the latter may be better understood and served.

Healing happens through letting go of what holds us back from being true to ourselves and our spiritual nature. Whether we have inherited inclinations from the past, such as addictive patterns of behaviour, experienced severe trauma during the journey from conception to birth, acquired a sense of abandonment during childhood or caused damage to ourselves or others during our adult lives, we need to allow ourselves to open up to what we are carrying within so that we can work through it and make amends where necessary. This process is set in motion most comprehensively by asking for compassion, firstly for oneself and then for those to whom we may have caused harm, so that whatever actions may follow are informed through the love and knowledge that unfolds through a spiritual perspective.

Developing the sense of spiritual awareness uncovers the knowledge that we emanate from a universal source of consciousness, in which the potential for healing is innate. The ability to access and work with the energy of healing is always available to everyone, according to their capacity to accept it. It is a universal invitation, offered without any condition other than the willingness to receive it, to serve it and to discover its possibilities in every being.

3.2

Healing Code of Honour

You are unique; just like everyone else.

ANON

Why is it necessary to consider a code of honour when working in healing and what does it mean to follow such a code? Whilst a code of conduct is a requirement formulated by professional bodies, to which practitioners are obliged to adhere, a personal code of honour goes beyond this in that it is an expression of one's individual integrity in the privacy of the relationship between practitioner and patient.

A personal code of honour is a reflection of the unique nature of this relationship which occurs in the intimacy of healing treatments, where the practitioner is present within the energy field of a patient. The integrity of a healing practitioner requires that they respect this completely, refraining from any interference or manipulation of the energy field during treatments.

The development of a personal code of honour will be unique to each practitioner. In looking at this it may be helpful to consider the following guidelines.

1 Be truthful to yourself and your goals.

2 Work unconditionally.

3 Resolve to fulfil your potential.

4 Understand the need for honesty in healing.

5 Maintain your patient's integrity.

6 Accept your past.

7 Honour yourself.

1 Be truthful to yourself and your goals

The adage 'know thyself' lies at the heart of the perennial teachings on wisdom and is as pertinent now as it always has been. Being involved with healing work necessarily brings up areas where one begins to see the restrictions and blockages in one's own energy field and how these have come about in the course of one's life. This is an integral part of our human nature. Anyone beginning to work in the healing field will find that certain matters will start to come to the surface and will require attention.

This process naturally involves the practitioner in a growing awareness of the importance of self-knowledge and of becoming a clearer place for the reception of healing energy. This cannot occur unless there is a commitment to this process, a willingness to learn from it and a determination to be guided by the truth inherent in every situation.

2 Work unconditionally

It is important to ensure that we do not bring any conditions into healing work, such as the expectation of a successful outcome of a treatment.

It is always helpful before starting a treatment to run a quick mental checklist to ensure one's intentions and motives are clear of personal attachments or desires which can colour the progress of the treatment. These can include a sense of personal ability as 'a healer', a desire to 'prove' that healing works, and the subconscious seeking of approval and self-validation. Such ego-driven considerations can be very subtle in their expression and we should always welcome any appearance of them as they present an opportunity for increased self-awareness and greater clarity in the responsibilities of healing work.

3 Resolve to fulfil your potential

Our potential lies hidden, waiting for expression. It is influenced by our genetic inheritance, our natural inclinations and tendencies, and by the accumulation of our life experiences. We become aware of what may be possible for us by exploring different interests and developing the skills which bring them into being. If we are drawn to healing work we need to be confident that all that is necessary for us to learn will be provided if we are prepared to follow the guidance that emerges from it.

We need to start with the affirmation that healing is possible, that we can engage in this work and that we can apply ourselves to learning all that is required to fulfil our potential in serving it.

4 Understand the need for honesty in healing

During healing work, situations may arise where it is necessary to speak about matters that could be difficult for the patient to hear. These can come about either through direct questions asked by the patient or through intuitive impressions and insights received by the practitioner.

Great sensitivity and tact are required on these occasions and the practitioner should always question whether or not it is necessary to impart such information and if so, what form it should take. It is essential to proceed with caution, but the practitioner always has a responsibility to adhere to the truth of what must be said. If this is denied or diluted then it may diminish the potential of the treatment to come to completion.

We may empathize with a patient and be reluctant to speak in a way that could cause distress; such reluctance, however, can act as a barrier in the treatment, obstructing its work. When it is necessary to communicate we always need to remember that our responsibility is to serve the real needs of the patient at the deepest level, balancing honesty with discretion and discernment, so that we may find the best arrangement in the words that are spoken.

We may be reluctant to hurt the feelings of another person, imagining how we would feel in their distress. Yet these very feelings may also act as an obstruction to the truth. As we grow in self-awareness so does our ability to discern what is a just cause and how best to serve the truth of the situation.

5 Maintain your patient's integrity

In healing work the relationship between practitioner and patient is intended to be one of intimacy and trust. In some situations, however, a patient may regard the practitioner as being an authority not only on healing, but, by extension, also on other areas of life. They may wish to relinquish their own personal responsibilities and attempt to involve the practitioner in making decisions, seeking their views and opinions.

A practitioner should always be aware of the possibility of this and refrain from accepting any position of influence over the patient.

6 Accept your past

If you are drawn to healing work it is important to follow it with determination and not to allow any difficult or past experiences to deflect you. It would be a mistake to think that anyone who wants to work in healing should be free of the past and any of its traumas before starting the process. Certainly these will need to be resolved, but in their proper time when the right help and guidance is available. Holding on to such memories can allow energy to be trapped, restricting what is possible in the present. It is helpful to recognize that being free from the past is a process which can take considerable time. By doing this, we do not cover up any difficulties; we acknowledge their existence but do not allow them to prevent us from moving forward.

7 Honour yourself

It is important in healing work to recognize that essentially we are not limited by time. That which we call 'spirit' is the real foundation of our existence and is timeless. This is our connection to the 'eternal' which takes us beyond all limitation and it is through this that 'healing' takes place. The more that we are receptive to this dimension within ourselves, by whatever name we call it, the more we allow it to manifest. To 'honour' this is to go beyond attachments of any kind and to relate to the reality in all living beings. It is this which we acknowledge both in ourselves and in our patients and only this which allows healing to be wholly present.

3.3

Professional Code of Practice

Know that a man may be very sincere in good
principles, without having good practice.

SAMUEL JOHNSON

Healing work involves two or more people who become as one for the duration of the healing process. What unites them is the act of healing itself, which gathers everyone involved into a circle of intimacy in which energy becomes activated by the requests and responses of the people involved. When energy is requested for the act of healing, it passes through the practitioner into the patient. The practitioner becomes a template so that the energy is directed clearly to where it needs to go; the less resistance there is to the flow of energy from the patient the more easily it will find its place. Equally, the less resistance there is from the practitioner, the more effective the act of healing becomes. The code of practice can be summarized as follows.

1 Always wait to be asked for healing.

2 Allow your intuition to be your guide.

3 Offer support without making promises.

4 Maintain confidentiality.

5 Ask for healing rather than treating yourself.

6   Preserve professional relationships with other healthcare practitioners.

7   Relate to healing, not to being a healer.

1 Always wait to be asked for healing

It is not advisable to offer healing, for in doing so the practitioner may interfere with a process that is taking place in the patient and prevent or distract it from its natural unfoldment. The act of healing seeks only to encourage the movement of energy, at whatever level is appropriate, in a spirit of co-operation between the patient and the practitioner. In certain situations however, for example in an emergency or when presented with a powerful intuitive request, it is necessary to ask for permission for healing from the patient's higher self, the reality which embraces all the levels of consciousness. If the answer is 'yes', then the healing may unfold; if it is 'no', then it is beneficial to send loving thoughts, as long as they are not conditioned in any way but sent for the sake of love itself.

2 Allow your intuition to be your guide

The intuitive faculty of consciousness goes to the heart of the matter. It is from here that guidance can be given for the act of healing to reach its full potential, directing the practitioner to the areas of the energy systems that need attention and to information that may or may not be shared with the patient. Without it the act of healing is only partial. Real intuition is always validated subsequently by other faculties of consciousness, such as intellect, confirming the insights given, regarding the patient's condition.

3 Offer support without making promises

The work of the healing practitioner is not to make promises about the future but to focus on the present. It is important to remember that the act of healing always begins in the present with the meeting of the patient and the practitioner. The practitioner's responsibility is to support the patient as they undergo the healing process, whether working internally in the energy field or through any discussions that may take place before, during or after the act of healing.

4 Maintain confidentiality

When a patient asks for healing and a practitioner accepts the request a bond of trust is forged between them. During the act of healing the practitioner enters the energy field of the patient and may receive insights which are intimate to the situation. Discussing these details with others, in whatever context, loosens and can break the bond, diminishing the effectiveness of any subsequent treatments. Should the treatments need to be discussed for the benefit of the patient, permission should always be sought first. In this way, the dignity of the patient is preserved and treatments may continue in an atmosphere of mutual respect.

5 Ask for healing rather than treating yourself

The act of healing involves three forces, the patient, the practitioner, and the potential for change which emerges from this creative exchange. If they become combined in one person, difficulties can often arise; without the mirror provided by the presence of another person the potential for the expression of energy is diminished. There is also an assumption of ability, that one can heal oneself through one's own power. In truth, healing takes place through the self but is not performed by it.

6 Preserve professional relationships with other healthcare practitioners

If problems arise from other medical or complementary therapies it is necessary to refer the patient back to the practitioner concerned. Practitioners are responsible for their own treatments, and to make comments concerning the work of others may confuse the patient and block the potential of the work in hand. It is beneficial to work in a spirit of co-operation with both complementary and conventional practitioners, since it expands the choices of effective healthcare, whereas conflict may constrict them. Each practice has its own rationale and validity and it is the responsibility of practitioners to give full measure in their treatments. Equally, it is the responsibility of patients to assess the results and to make the ultimate decisions that relate to their own well-being.

7 Relate to healing, not to being a healer

One should be very careful of becoming attached to the gift of healing and of taking it to oneself. It is necessary to remember that it is a gift which is only given to allow one to be of service to healing. It is not a gift that can be possessed or limited. If there is attachment to being a 'healer' stagnation may occur, preventing a practitioner developing, both professionally and in other areas of life. Any successful outcomes in healing treatments are by virtue of the power of healing itself, which is channelled through but not determined by the practitioner.

The Practitioner–Patient Relationship

The relationship between the patient and the practitioner begins in the present but may often involve details of past experiences and future expectations which can prevent a patient from focusing on what is real in the moment. Patients may often arrive with specific illnesses or problems by which they may define themselves. The practitioner needs to go beyond this and relate to the potential for healing for the whole person.

In order to do this, firstly it is helpful to go beyond any reactions, positive or negative, with regard to a patient. There are some people to whom we relate more easily than others, and some with whom we may feel uncomfortable. In this situation we should look into ourselves to see why we respond in this way. Such reactions may be the projection of an inner state of unresolved conflict, often reaching back into childhood or adolescence. By facing these feelings, the underlying reasons for them can emerge. Through the insights given to us, reaction may be transformed into reflection so that we become opened to a more generous and pragmatic perspective.

It is important for healing practitioners to focus their sensitivities and skills within themselves as well as with their patients. The more willing they are to do this, the better they are able to support them through the healing process. At the heart of this is a belief and trust that we have the resources within us which will draw out an increased self-awareness.

Healing takes place at a profound level where a patient may experience an acceptance which is completely unconditioned. This is an attractive and contagious state, but if it is attached to a practitioner it alters the nature of the relationship. It can produce a womb-like condition in which the patient embeds in the energy field of the practitioner, seeking their solace and sustenance from there. Its existence may be necessary for a period of time but the objective of the practitioner is to encourage each patient to find an individual inner source of strength and purpose.

Within the attachment lies its means of release, which will make itself known when the time is right. If it is addressed when the timing is wrong, the patient may feel bereft and abandoned by the person in whom so much trust and dependence has been placed, and seek to find another womb, since the inner focus required for self-responsibility has yet to be established.

On some occasions a healing 'crisis' arises from the treatment when the symptoms of disease are released from the body rather than being absorbed by it.

Healing can produce major symptoms rather than side effects, as it works directly on the energy systems. These may take the form of physical or psychological pain, and a temporary feeling of exhaustion may overwhelm the patient after the release of long-standing and powerfully restrained tensions. It is important for the practitioner to explain to the patient that this may occur. Should it happen, the practitioner needs to identify what is taking place and recognize that this is part of a known condition described as 'the law of cure', rather than any deficiency in the treatment or in the patient's response to it.

Going through the law of cure of the healing crisis is a different experience from becoming ill. Whilst the latter feels like 'going down' with an illness, the former feels like 'coming up' from it, discharging any remaining traces of it along the way. This is often experienced as a sense of clearing and may require further support, either through more healing or in conversation.

3.3

Conversation Skills

Strangers talk; friends listen.

ANON

Conversation literally means 'to turn with'. In real conversation there is both speaking and listening, the topics turning with the momentum of what is being said. One-sided conversation, which is talking at the other person rather than discussing with them, occurs when the speaker is concerned only with their own point of view or assumes a position of influence over the listener. This may manifest as:

◆ advice: 'If I were you I'd ...'

◆ sympathy: 'It must be so awful for you ...'

◆ self-disclosure: 'I must tell you what happened to me when ...'

◆ guidance: 'Now you must be positive ...'

These words assume that the speaker knows what is best for the listener. In healing treatments it is fundamental for the practitioner to work *with* a patient to explore a problem and seek an outcome. This is much more effective than dispensing advice which can overwhelm patients and make it harder for them to take responsibility for their problems.

Patients may appreciate sympathy from a practitioner but this is limited in its effect – they benefit more from an empathetic approach which helps them go beyond self-concern in order to find a wider and more objective perspective of their situation, becoming proactive in the process. There may be occasions when an example from a practitioner's own experience can be of help to a patient. Such self-disclosure should be very carefully considered and only used when completely relevant.

Urging a patient to change their state of mind is rarely productive. Recommendations such as 'You must be positive' are ignoring the reality of how the patient is and imposing a particular point of view which prevents the patient from asserting his or her own needs.

Two-sided conversation requires a balance of speaking and listening, so that there is a natural flow between the two. Within this there is the willingness to listen and not interrupt until the speaker is finished, so that whatever needs to be said can unfold in full measure. When the speaker is free to speak and the listener to listen, then communication really begins.

Communication takes many forms, in which speaking may play only a small part. It is vital to observe the effects of conversation through the responses of the body and in what is left unsaid. If there are strong feelings that are not expressed, such as anger or depression, they can inhibit the flow of the conversation. Whilst recognizing these, it is better that they remain unspoken until the patient is ready to reveal them. Signs that the patient finds the conversation too difficult to continue include fidgeting, sitting on the edge of the seat, and avoiding eye contact, all of which indicate that the connection between practitioner and patient is weakening. If the patient becomes repetitive without moving forward, so that he or she continually revolves around the same point, the practitioner needs to refocus the dialogue by introducing appropriate questions. If at this point the conversation cannot be retrieved it is best to conclude it until the next meeting.

Attentiveness is important in ensuring that authentic communication takes place. Being attentive means not thinking about anything other than what is being said, whilst it is being said. An understanding of what is being said comes simply from a way of listening that concentrates on the words as they are being spoken.

Pausing provides time for both parties to think about what has been said, and to respond as necessary. When pauses are allowed to happen naturally in conversation they help to score the the rhythm and pace of it, directing attention to both the spoken and unspoken elements of dialogue. Silence can create an atmosphere of acceptance, which can give the speaker the courage to reveal their innermost thoughts.

These four guidelines for authentic conversation can be remembered by using the following acronym:

S – Space

O – Observation

A – Attention

P – Pause

As in 'Always use SOAP'.

There are occasions when the patient may need to speak for a considerable length of time, either before or after receiving healing: indeed the words released can often become part of the healing process. The patient may need to ask questions before the treatment and to discuss the effects of it afterwards. In these instances it is advisable to go into 'healing mode' so that the practitioner's own energy is not drawn upon, and both have access to the limitless source of energy from the universal healing consciousness. There are four steps into 'healing mode', which are:

G – Grounding

A – Attunement

P – Protection

P – Permission

As in 'Mind the GAPP'.

Being grounded in the physical body allows an anchoring for genuine conversation to take place, since all the senses are accessed. Attunement to the healing energy enables consciousness to use all its faculties. Protection prevents personal energy from being drawn out of either the practitioner or the patient. Permission for the work to happen allows the intimacy of healing to begin.

When the practitioner and the patient are united in the same field of universal healing energy, an internal conversation may occur. This is a dialogue in the language of energy, as it expresses itself through the body processes, the meridians, the chakras and the aura. This may appear in the form of colours, images or words that convey meaning which deepens understanding. Similarly, the patient may engage in an inner dialogue with what is happening inside their body, as a result of the healing work that is taking place.

This is the conversation of healing, sometimes called the language of the heart. When words are spoken from there, they have the ability to dissolve conflict and create harmony.

Conversation Skills: Practical Exercise

1 Sit quietly and take a few deep breaths to prepare to enter into the consciousness of healing by using the following technique.

Mind the GAPP

Grounding: Ask to be still in your body so that you feel connected to the earth through your feet.

Attunement: Ask to be focused in your mind so that you can be receptive to the consciousness of the universal healing energy which is ever present and accessible.

Protection: Ask for your own personal energy to be preserved. Imagine yourself surrounded by a globe of white light to ensure that you do not draw from your own energy during the healing.

Permission: Ask for consent to be given from the patient for the healing work to take place.

Always use SOAP

Space: Listen to your patient without interrupting.

Observation: Observe body language and respond accordingly.

Attention: Concentrate on what is being said and also what the meaning is behind the words.

Pause: Before following up on what has been said allow time for reflection. Seek to mirror, not to guide.

2 Practise listening to another person for a few minutes and interrupt several times. Then repeat the exercise, listening without interrupting.

3   Practise speaking to another person, but have them interrupting you several
    times. Then practise speaking without their interrupting you.

4   Give honest feedback to one another about the results of this exercise.

3.5

The Breath

Student, tell me where is God?

It is the breath inside the breath.

KABIR

Our life begins and ends with breath, which encapsulates the power that keeps us alive. It holds the life force which is transmitted through the breath into the blood where it is transported it into every cell of the body.

We inhale air and exhale carbon dioxide through the action of the lungs and the diaphragm – the sheet of smooth dome-shaped muscle that contracts on inhalation and causes exhalation when it relaxes. The breath acts as a link between mind and body; this is clearly demonstrated in practices such as yoga and t'ai chi and in the change of state which always results from conscious breathing exercises. Becoming conscious of one's breath helps to develop awareness of the state of the body and the mind. Breathing practices can develop sensitivity both in oneself and when working with others. They can help to ground the body and focus the mind so that concentration can be sustained not only in healing, but in any situation.

Whilst the action of the breath is governed by the autonomic nervous system, it can be controlled to some extent by breathing exercises, for example in preparation for the practice of meditation.

The Breath: Practical Exercise

Practise deep breathing:

- into the throat;
- into the chest;
- into the abdomen.

How to breathe deeply:

- Hold your chin up.
- Keep your shoulders back.
- Keep your back straight.
- Stand with your feet slightly apart.
- Take a breath through your nose to a count of 7 seconds.
- Allow your abdomen to extend outwards.
- Hold your breath for a count of 28 seconds.
- Release your breath through your nose to a count of 14 seconds.
- Allow your abdomen to contract.
- Sit quietly.
- Allow your energy to settle.
- Check that you feel grounded
- Record any impressions that you may have received

If the breath count is too high for you, lower it, whilst working with ratio of 1:4:2 for inhaling: holding: exhaling.

3.6

Meditation

In meditation go deep in the heart;
In action watch the timing.

LAO TSU

To engage in meditation is to deepen the relationship with oneself, and to observe what is happening through the power of contemplative thought. It is an invitation to withdraw into the inner sanctum of one's being. Meditation is guided by intention, commitment and concentration. Intention is needed to start the practice, commitment to follow it and concentration to give oneself wholly to it.

The practice of meditation may help to sharpen the physical senses, clear the mind and connect us with the unconditioned and timeless nature of our real being. It is beneficial both in daily life and specifically in healing practice because it allows access to those deeper levels of consciousness which may come into view during treatments. It is also helpful for practitioners to allow some contemplative time for themselves on a regular basis. Meditation encourages us to explore and develop our inner resources and to establish a grounded and centred connection to our daily life.

Practical Exercise: Introduction to Meditation

Allow a time when you are not likely to be disturbed and give yourself between 10 and 30 minutes for this practice. Use a watch or a timer if you prefer. If you follow it regularly, choose the same time each day.

+ Sit quietly.

+ Breathe deeply and evenly.

+ Observe the rising and falling of your breath.

+ Be aware of any tensions or worries within you.

+ Allow them to leave on the out-breath.

+ Breathe in peace on the in-breath.

+ Follow the flow of your breathing. If thoughts or images arise do not allow them to distract you; return your attention to the breath.

When it is time to finish the meditation take a short period to:

+ bring your consciousness into the present,

+ feel your body earthed through your feet, and

+ conclude the meditation.

Guided Meditation

In guided meditation, a map is provided to direct and focus the mind on its journey into deeper levels of consciousness. This map may be composed of sounds, as in music, of objects, such as icons, and words, as used in prayers or mantras.

There are three guided meditations provided here which use creative visualization to support the work of healing, for practitioners and patients alike.

The first one, 'Visiting Your Healing Place' is used to gain insight into personal health, and may be used as often as necessary.

'Untying the Knots that Bind' helps release long held and deeply felt emotional distress. This should be used cautiously and often in conjunction with therapeutic support to complete the healing process.

'Acknowledging Presences of Help' recognizes the timeless nature of healing work, and may be used in healing training and practice.

Visiting your Healing Place

This guided meditation proposes the presence of a setting that is uniquely designed and supplied with whatever is required to support your well-being. It is your own personalized health centre, which offers guidance through the five senses of the body and the five faculties of the mind.

- ◆ Sit quietly.

- ◆ Take some sighing breaths.

- ◆ If you wish, take a few deep breaths.

- ◆ Ask for your consciousness to take you to your healing place.

- ◆ Allow yourself to be guided to wherever you need to go.

- ◆ When you arrive in your healing place allow your senses and faculties to discover what is there.

- ◆ What can you see, hear, touch, smell, taste?

- ◆ What is your instinctive response to these senses?

- ◆ What do you feel?

- ◆ What are you thinking?

- ◆ Where does your imagination take you?

- ◆ What is your intuitive response?

- ◆ Find somewhere in your healing place where you can relax and absorb whatever information came to you.

- ◆ When the work is done and you are ready to leave, give thanks for anything you have received.

- ◆ Ask for your consciousness to take you back the way you came and return you to the present moment.

- ◆ Check that you are grounded in body and settled in mind.

Untying the Knots that Bind

These knots appear as blocks in the energy field which may affect physical health through illness and so-called accidental injuries, and psychological health through neuroses and psychotic conditions. When we are born we bring with us the imprints of past generations through our genetic inheritance. Some of them are beneficial whilst others may be constrictive or harmful. These remain with us until they are recognized, addressed and dispersed, often with therapeutic help. Further imprints come into play during the passage of life itself, some of which may have an adverse effect on our health and our capacity to fulfil our potential.

To have these negative imprints released allows trapped energy to flow properly so that not only is health improved, but also our latent abilities may be expressed more completely.

◆ Sit quietly.

◆ Take some sighing breaths.

◆ If you wish, take one or two deep breaths.

◆ Ask for your consciousness to take you to a place of healing where you may be freed from attachments that you no longer need.

◆ Wait quietly so that any thoughts or images may arise in their own time.

◆ Witness your thoughts and impressions without trying to alter them in any way.

◆ If memories come to mind stay with them and reflect on their meaning:

   – What is there to learn from them?

   – Are there any apologies to be made to anyone for past actions? These may be made in person and if that is not possible then by the power of thought, so that apologies may be transmitted to wherever they need to go.

   – Are there any apologies to be received by you from people in the past who may appear in the mind's eye during the meditation? Such a person may be from the distant past and unknown to you. Should this happen, allow whatever is necessary to unfold so that you do not prevent any apologies from being made.

   – Are there impressions received that allow a clearer insight into the present?

   – Are there insights to be gained that will help guide the way into the future?

◆ Allow yourself to be released from attachments that you no longer need.

- When the work is done and you are ready to leave your healing place give thanks for anything you have received.
- Ask for your consciousness to take you back the way you came and return you to the present moment.
- Check that you are grounded in body and settled in mind.

Acknowledging Presences of Help

Healing is transmitted through the power of thought, which is instigated through request. It is important in the act of healing that we ask to be a clear channel, so that whatever is transmitted through us is not affected by the personal self, but is true to the healing itself.

During this process of transmission the practitioner may become aware of the presence of others.

It should be understood that part of the healing process can at times involve connection with other levels of existence from which guidance and help are available. These presences may be sensed, seen through clairvoyance, heard through clairaudience or experienced as forms of light. Their presence may become clearer and stronger during the act of healing. If this is experienced it is not necessary for the practitioner to engage with them. Their function is to be of service in the healing. It is sufficient to acknowledge them and continue with the treatment.

This guided meditation for practitioners may be used in training programmes with those interested in learning about healing work. It can increase awareness of the deeper levels of consciousness through which such help may appear.

- Sit quietly.
- Take some sighing breaths.
- If you wish, take one or two deep breaths.
- Ask to be taken to the levels of existence in which these presences of help are accessible
- Allow yourself to be guided to wherever you need to go.
- When you arrive at your destination, ask to be cleansed in mind and body through the light of the healing consciousness.
- Ask to be connected with those healing presences who are completely attuned to the energy of healing consciousness.

- ◆ Stay with them until it is time for you to go.
- ◆ When you are ready to leave give thanks for what you have received.
- ◆ Ask to be returned through your consciousness to the present moment.
- ◆ Check that you are grounded in body and settled in mind.

3.7

Grounding

If you are rooted in the ground
your arms may reach to heaven.

ANON

Grounding is essential during the act of healing, so that the practitioner is fully present with the patient and able to observe any changes that are taking place. Being grounded makes us acutely aware of our surroundings, through all the senses of the body and faculties of the mind.

It is preferable for the practitioner to keep their eyes open as much as possible during this time so that they do not enter into a state of trance, which would disconnect them from the immediacy of the treatment. It may also be helpful to remove footwear so that the direct contact of the feet with the floor earths their energy field.

A practitioner who is grounded is centred within the consciousness of healing with all seven levels of energy in alignment with one another, so that there is a clear channel through which the act of healing may take place.

Experiencing Grounding by Working Through the Chakras

Focus your energy on each chakra in turn.

Crown	How open do you feel when you are grounded?
Brow	How do your thoughts appear to you when you are grounded?

Throat	Can drinking water help you to feel more grounded?
Heart	How do you relate to yourself when you are grounded?
Solar plexus	How does it feel to be grounded?
Sacral	How do you relate to others when you are grounded?
Base	How do you make a connection to the earth?

Practising Grounding

♦ Perform a simple ablution, using water if possible; if it is not available, ask to be cleansed by healing energy.

♦ Sit quietly.

♦ Take some sighing breaths.

♦ If you wish, take one or two deep breaths.

♦ Ask to be brought into the present moment; allow thoughts that dwell in the past or speculate on the future to float away, and ask to be returned to the present moment.

♦ Breathe slowly and gently and allow the moments within the breaths to unfold.

♦ Give thanks for your experience of grounding.

♦ Record any information that may be helpful to you.

3.8

Attunement

The inward being is not at all in time or place,
but is purely and simply in eternity.

MEISTER ECKHART

Attunement takes place when the practitioner adjusts to the energy of the universal healing consciousness.

It is accepted by many involved in medicine that there is a presence of healing, a state of consciousness that gives exactly what is required to bring about harmony, provided that the right conditions have been established. These conditions require the patient to be as relaxed as possible, willing to allow the necessary changes to take place.

The process of attunement has been compared to tuning into a radio station, although in the case of healing the information is heard by the inner rather than the outer ear. It demands stillness and concentration. The former is required to bring the practitioner into the present, which gives access to deeper levels of consciousness, and the latter guides the mind to the intention of healing, enabling the practitioner to understand what needs to take place.

With practice, we can become attuned swiftly to the presence of healing. It may take place through prayer, deep breathing techniques, or other means which present themselves to the consciousness of the healing practitioner. When attunement occurs, the crown chakra opens to allow healing energy to be transmitted from the practitioner to the patient. If this produces any sensations of discomfort or disharmony it may be necessary to protect this chakra from external influences by commanding it to close and by asking for the healing energies to be directed through the brow chakra. The area between the crown and the brow then remains the private domain of the practitioner, protected from both the exterior forces of the environment and the patient's physical, psychological and spiritual states.

Working through either the crown or the brow chakra in all the faculties of consciousness allows the process of attunement to direct the healing as it wills, establishing the order and pattern of the treatment.

Experiencing Attunement by Working Through the Chakras

Focus your energy on each chakra.

Crown	What sensations do you experience when your crown chakra is open through the five senses (hearing, sight, smell, taste and touch)?
Brow	Observe your thoughts as they arise through the five faculties (instinct, feelings, intellect, imagination, and intuition).
Throat	Take some deep breaths to reinvigorate yourself.
Heart	Allow the effects of the breathing to settle.
Solar plexus	Let your feelings ebb and flow. Don't engage with them as they pass through the seat of your emotions.
Sacral	Create time for yourself as you would with someone you care for.
Base	Ground yourself in the present and make your request for attunement.

Practising Attunement

◆ Perform a simple ablution, using water if possible; if it is not available ask to be cleansed by healing energy.

◆ Sit quietly.

◆ Take some sighing breaths.

◆ If you wish, take some deep breaths.

◆ Ask to be attuned to the energy of the universal healing consciousness.

◆ Observe the sensations that arise and allow them to flow without interference.

◆ Give thanks for the experience of attunement that you have received.

◆ Record any information that may be helpful to you.

3.9

Protection

To maintain your centre is to endure.

LAO TSU

Protection is vital in the act of healing to ensure that the practitioner and the patient do not exchange personal energies with one another. The practitioner is required to become a clear channel for the energy of the universal healing consciousness, and the patient to become receptive to it. This happens through request, when the patient asks for healing and the practitioner asks for protection. A circle of healing energy is created, enclosing both practitioner and patient, which enables the work to happen within a protective boundary, containing the flow of energy and directing it to where it needs to go. When the work has been completed the boundaries may be dissolved, again through request, leaving both practitioner and patient within their own centres of energy. At this point they have been removed from the protection that is given during the act of healing but may call upon its power if the need arises again during their time together.

It is necessary for all of us, whether we are involved with the care of others or not, to understand the need for personal protection. If we do not preserve our energy boundaries we leave ourselves open to invasion by energy from elsewhere. The effects of this can vary from the mild to the extreme. Carrying energy which is not our own can reveal itself at one end of the spectrum as discomfort or unexplained distress, and at the other as obsessive thoughts about people or situations and extreme reactions to them. In the past this situation was sometimes regarded as possession; it can still be described as having inner demons, but also as internalizing someone else's negative state.

The practice of ablution, the saying of prayers, and the act of healing can be effective in clearing the energy field of invasive forces so that it is free to be itself again. Ablution not only physically cleanses the person or the place where negativity is felt, but also helps to clear the psychological state and prevent negativity from returning. Prayers carry a powerful presence through the recital of their words, and their purity can dissolve negativity. The act of healing provides the conditions for this energy to be expelled and revives the existing energy as necessary.

We live in a world of energy exchange that is a continuous cycle of absorption and release. Within this setting it is vital for us to preserve a sense of self. Doing so allows us a connection with our own feelings and experiences which can guide us to live according to our own frame of reference, whilst being open to, but not becoming entangled by, what is going on in other people's lives.

Healthcare practitioners can be susceptible to ill health because their work takes them into the energy field of their patients, especially when it involves touch. If healing practitioners don't ask for protection then their own energy will be used in the healing process. While there is an endless abundance of the universal healing energy, our own is confined to our bodies. We can develop powerful energy fields, which attract the attention of those in need; where energy is weak it will seek a source of strength to replenish it. If our own energy fields are unprotected our crown chakras will open to the instinctive request for healing from those in distress. When the crown chakra remains open permanently it can lead to a debilitating state of physical, psychological and spiritual exhaustion, that prohibits further healing work from taking place.

When our own personal energy is drawn from us it can leave us feeling very weak, light-headed or nauseous and reluctant to carry out familiar tasks. It can take several hours or even longer for energy to replenish itself, although a healing treatment may speed up the process. It is necessary to be aware of the warning signs that show that energy is being drawn from you. These may include sensations in the chakras, especially in the crown, the heart or the solar plexus. Once these are recognized, protection can be put in place immediately through asking for it to be given in whatever form is most appropriate.

Healing practitioners may also be affected if they do not allow enough time for themselves. The needs of others can become so absorbing and demanding that they leave little time and space for their own requirements. Practising the art of healing can enhance sensitivity beyond the healing circle of the treatment room into daily life. We should be aware of how we respond to people in need so that healing is never given unless it is requested, otherwise it will interfere with the integrity of both the practitioner and the patient.

Protection should become a daily practice; not done in an obsessive manner nor out of constriction but out of value for oneself, as a sensible and natural precaution.

Practical Guidelines for Energy Invasion

Causes

- ◆ Disconnection from one's own feelings, needs and experiences.
- ◆ Overabsorption with the life of another person or lives of other people.
- ◆ A misplaced sense of responsibility in response towards other people's problems.
- ◆ The power of negative or hostile thought.

Signs and Symptoms

- ◆ Feeling tired and drained.
- ◆ Feeling burdened by daily living.
- ◆ Feeling another 'presence' continually.
- ◆ Feeling negative towards oneself, in the extreme, to the extent of self-loathing, or feeling suicidal.
- ◆ Taking on a different persona.
- ◆ Exaggerated or destructive behaviour.
- ◆ Recurrent illnesses of an unexplained nature, e.g. 'psychotic episodes'.
- ◆ Injuries of unexplained nature.

Treatment

◆ Ablution.

◆ Saying of prayers.

◆ Use of crystals in dowsing for blocked energy.

◆ Sprinkling of sweet water (i.e. water containing sugar).

◆ Command: 'If anyone, anywhere is sending me anything good or bad, I send it back.'

◆ Distant or contact healing.

Experiencing Protection by Working Through the Chakras

Focus your energy on each chakra.

Crown	Open up to the meaning of protection and where it is necessary in your life.
Brow	Set the intention for meditation so that you can observe your state of mind and how it needs to protect itself.
Throat	Use your voice in prayers of your choice, mantras, and chanting to invoke the protective power of the spoken word.
Heart	Examine how you feel when you experience the security of protection in your daily life, in healthcare and in healing.
Solar plexus	Examine how you feel when your sense of security is threatened in your daily life, in healthcare and in healing.
Sacral	Work with your imagination to create images of protection.
Base	Be mindful of your needs for energy protection in crowds, threatening situations, with needy people and during healing treatments.

Practising Protection

- ◆ Perform a simple ablution, using water if possible; if it is not available, ask to be cleansed by healing energy.

- ◆ Sit quietly.

- ◆ Take some sighing breaths.

- ◆ If you wish, take some deep breaths.

- ◆ Ask yourself how you may best be protected: allow thoughts and images to come to mind and ask to be guided to what will work most effectively for you.

- ◆ Give thanks for the experience of protection which you have been given.

- ◆ Record anything that may be helpful to you.

3.10

Permission

Ask and it shall be given you.

MATTHEW 7:7

Permission is essential for the act of healing, so that it takes place in a hospitable environment. When permission to enter the energy field of another for the purpose of healing is not sought it may be likened to entering someone else's home without their agreement.

By asking for permission for the work of healing to take place we acknowledge that we do not have the power to heal others, but that we are in service to the reality of healing, which expresses itself with a range and depth far beyond conditioned human comprehension.

If permission is not granted, because the patient has changed their mind, expressing themselves verbally or through their intuitive voice which is heard by the practitioner, the act of healing should not take place. It may be replaced with a period of relaxation or conversation and set in motion again when the patient is ready to receive the universal healing energy that is channelled through the practitioner.

Asking for permission for healing to take place is an act of tact, an expression of spiritual good manners. Once granted, the need for permission continues throughout the exchange. Permission may be sought internally again during the healing, as a reminder of its importance in establishing a good relationship between the practitioner and patient, so that nothing takes place energetically without full agreement.

Experiencing Permission by Working Through the Chakras

Focus your energy on each chakra.

Crown	Allow your crown chakra to open up into healing mode.
Brow	Reflect on what the word permission means to you.
Throat	Seek the correct words for you to use when asking for permission to go into healing mode.
Heart	How do you give yourself your permission?
Solar plexus	How does it make you feel when you grant yourself permission?
Sacral	How do good manners relate to permission in your relationships with others?
Base	How do good manners relate to permission in the world which you create for yourself?

Practising Permission

- Perform a simple ablution, using water if possible; if it is not available, ask to be cleansed by healing energy.

- Sit quietly.

- Take some sighing breaths.

- If you wish, take some deep breaths.

- Ask for permission to be in service to the work of healing.

- Allow thoughts and images to come to mind and let them inform you about what it means to be of service in this work.

- Give thanks for your experience.

- Record anything that may helpful to you.

3.11

Sensing Energy

Earth cannot show so brave a sight
As when a single soul does fence
The batteries of alluring sense
And Heaven views it with delight.

ANDREW MARVELL,
DIALOGUE BETWEEN THE RESOLVED SOUL AND CREATED PLEASURE

Everyone has their own way of sensing energy. It may be through vision, touch, images, thoughts, words or pressure. Some practitioners only sense energy intuitively without any specific form. What is important when learning about healing is not to have expectations or to make comparisons with other students. A person may be drawn to one or a number of ways of sensing energy. It is necessary for each to follow what is best for them and to develop their own particular way of working.

The energy surrounding every living being may be experienced through the five senses. These senses are reflected in the five elements of nature. The energy in our bodies is generated by the external environment and the food we eat. According to the five elements law of acupuncture the seasons of nature (Spring, Summer, Late Summer, Autumn and Winter) are associated with the elements of wood, fire, earth, metal and water.

- ◆ Spring resonates to the element of wood, which activates new growth.

◆ Summer resonates to the element of fire, which spreads the growth.

◆ Late Summer resonates to the element of earth, which stabilizes the growth.

◆ Autumn resonates to the element of metal, which inhibits further growth.

◆ Winter resonates to the element of water, which contains the moisture required for the Spring.

Following the guidelines of the five elements, as shown in figure 27, enables us to detect energy through our senses. It takes both study and practice to hear the tone of the voice, to observe the hue coming from the skin, to smell the odour emanating from the body, and to investigate taste through food preference and the patient's 'taste' for life. The process gives us not only a deeper sense of others but also of ourselves.

Each element is also associated with the meridians as outlined below:

Element	Meridians
Wood	Liver and gall bladder
Fire	Heart, heart protector, small intestine and triple heater
Earth	Spleen and stomach
Metal	Lungs and large intestine
Water	Kidneys and bladder

The meridians may be sensed through the fingers and toes, each of which relate to a specific channel of energy and the flow of energy that begins or ends in them. The two vessels can be felt either side of the hand, the governor on the outer and the conception on the inner. The meridians may also be sensed at the junction points along the energy pathways, all of which have a psychological as well as a physical function. The more we learn about the language of the meridians, the more insights may be gained into the patient's physical, psychological and spiritual health.

Figure 27: Sensing energy through the five elements

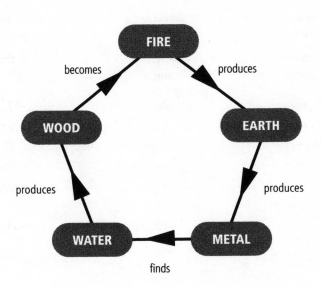

Sensing the elements

Season	Elements	Colour	Sound	Smell	Taste	Touch
Spring	Wood	Green	Shouting	Rancid	Sour	Dense
Summer	Fire	Red	Laughing	Acrid	Bitter	Hot
Late Summer	Earth	Yellow	Humming	Fragrant	Sweet	Cool
Autumn	Metal	White	Crying	Fishy	Spicy	Damp
Winter	Water	Black	Groaning	Rotten	Salty	Cold

Figure 28: Sensing the energy of the meridians in the hands and the feet

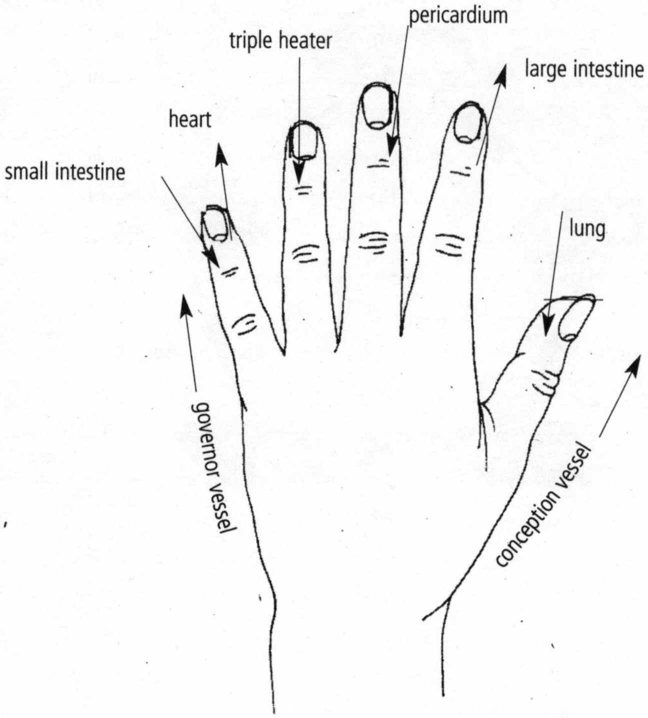

triple heater

pericardium

large intestine

heart

small intestine

lung

governor vessel

conception vessel

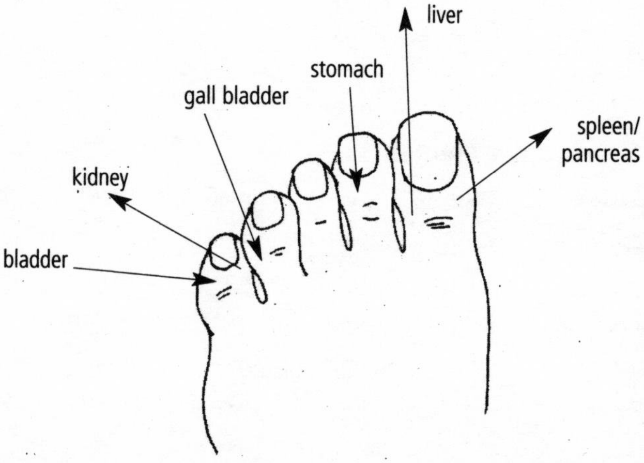

liver

stomach

gall bladder

spleen/ pancreas

kidney

bladder

The direction of the arrows indicates whether the flow of energy begins or ends in the fingers or toes

When working with the meridians in the context of spiritual healing it is important to remember that they should not be manipulated in any way. The work of healing happens when the relevant energies are activated and begin to reformulate themselves. They may be witnessed by the practitioner, and felt by the patient, as energy flows to or from the hands or the feet. This is an indication that the work is taking place throughout the network of channels, but without any assistance in the form of needles, herbs or pressure.

Similarly, the energy of the chakras may be sensed when the hands are placed near them. The practitioner should allow the information contained in the energy to express itself in circular movements of varying intensity through the palms of the hands or the soles of the feet. The lower chakras: the base, the sacral and the solar plexus often feel more dense, as they vibrate at a slower rate than the upper ones: the throat, the brow and the crown, which are finer and lighter, and vibrate at a higher rate. Situated at the midpoint, the heart chakra co-ordinates all the others and may also be sensed through the radial pulses in both wrists. One should let the hands be guided by the information from the chakras as to how long to remain in contact with them and when to move on.

Within the context of spiritual healing it is vital when working with the chakras to start from the crown and work downwards to the base. If work begins at the base it can circulate toxic energies which may have accumulated there into the whole system and may cause profound damage in the physical, psychological and spiritual levels of consciousness.

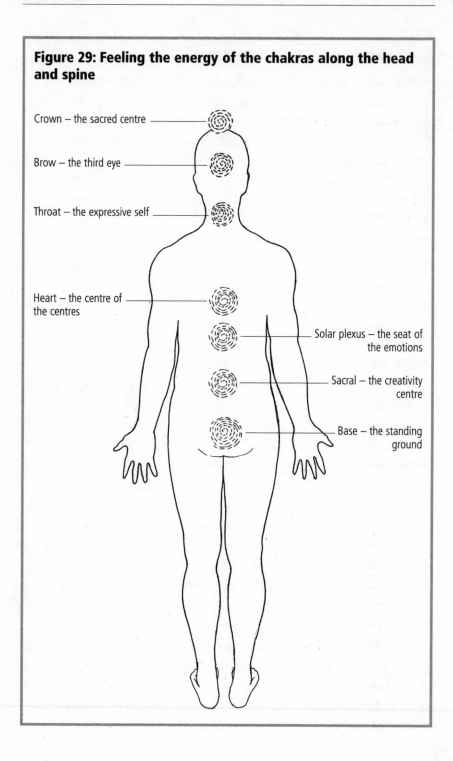

Figure 29: Feeling the energy of the chakras along the head and spine

Crown – the sacred centre

Brow – the third eye

Throat – the expressive self

Heart – the centre of the centres

Solar plexus – the seat of the emotions

Sacral – the creativity centre

Base – the standing ground

Colours that may be observed in the aura

Colour	Light	Bright	Dark
Red	Weak	Vigorous	Angry
Orange	Cautious	Cheerful	Confused
Yellow	Dreamy	Stimulating	Dogmatic
Green	Passive	Harmonious	Envious
Turquoise	Uncommunicative	Eloquent	Repetitive
Blue	Reactive	Reflective	Resistant
Purple – white	Drained	Cleansed	Congested

There are two ways of looking at the aura. One occurs naturally when colours are seen around the patient's body. Otherwise the practitioner should enter into a healing mode of grounding, attunement, permission and protection. Consciousness is then placed in their inner or third eye located in the brow chakra in the middle of the forehead. From this the practitioner looks through the patient and may see the colours of the patient's aura reflected on the wall. Colours may appear, as though on a screen, in a myriad of images, weaving threads of energy into shape and form. These colours relate to all the bodies of the energy field. If sensed through the hands, they manifest as a force, or a pressure, which prevents the hands from moving closer to the owner of the aura. The substance of the pressure may feel almost like rubber; there is some give in it but also a powerful inner resistance.

The colours of the aura reflect the energy responses in the human being. These colours are ever moving and during the act of healing may be seen to rearrange themselves, merging in and out of each other, until they vibrate with a greater sense of harmony.

Being sensitive to energy allows the practitioner to understand more about how it works in the structures and functions of the body and how to explore its relationship with the meridians and the chakras.

This understanding can also deepen the connection with the practitioner's own body so that they are more aware of how the energy responds both to internal and external influences. It also helps to develop a real appreciation of the 'intelligence' which is expressed through the flow of energy in the organization and detailing of life throughout all levels of existence.

Practice of Healing: Sensing Energy
Preparation
For this exercise you will need to work with a partner. Ensure that your partner is comfortable. Practice some relaxation techniques if necessary.

Open up into 'Healing Mode'
Connect to your healing consciousness through:

Grounding: Ask to be present in your body.

Attunement: Ask to be linked in mind to the energy of healing consciousness.

Protection: Ask for protection for your personal energy.

Permission: Ask to be allowed to sense energy.

The Meridians
For this exercise your partner should be sitting down whilst you face them.

◆ Place your hands over your partner's fingers and then toes.

◆ Record any sensations that you may experience in your fingers or toes, or in any other part of your body.

◆ Share any sensations that you experience.

The Chakras
For this exercise your partner should be sitting down.

◆ Stand behind your partner whilst you are opening up into the healing mode.

◆ Use your intuition to select which chakra to work with.

◆ Now stand at one side. Place both hands with fingers apart on either side of the chakra at the front and back of the body, but not touching it.

◆ Observe any sensations that you may feel in the palms of your hands, the soles of your feet or any other part of the body.

◆ Share any sensations that you experienced if appropriate.

The Aura

For this exercise your partner should be sitting down with their back against a plain wall.

- ◆ Place your consciousness in the inner, or third eye, located in the brow chakra.

- ◆ Look through your brow chakra into and beyond the patient's brow chakra and focus on the wall behind them.

- ◆ Allow images and insights to unfold from your inner and outer senses.

- ◆ Share your images and insights if appropriate.

Closing Down from 'Healing Mode'

Permission: Give thanks for the agreement that has been received and for the healing that has taken place.

Protection: Ask to be returned to your personal circle of energy.

Attunement: Ask to be present in mind.

Grounding: Ask to be present in body.

3.12

Preparation for the Act of Healing

Without preparation there will be no beginning.

ANON

There are seven steps to take in preparation for the act of healing, which may be referred to as the seven 'C's', and which relate in their function to the chakras.

1 Communication

2 Code of conduct

3 Calmness

4 Clothing

5 Channelling

6 Crisis

7 Comfort

1 Being ready to communicate involves:

- ◆ having immediate access to your appointment diary;
- ◆ speaking in a direct and friendly way when using the telephone;
- ◆ providing business cards, leaflets and location maps;
- ◆ being available to give talks and work at exhibitions;
- ◆ creating a website;

- placing advertisements and writing articles for newspapers and magazines; and

- providing information on research and anecdotal evidence in healing.

2 Applying your code of conduct involves:

- setting the intention to honour your code of conduct both personally and professionally;

- formulating and respecting your personal code of conduct;

- integrating your professional code of conduct in your healing practice;

- questioning your professional code of conduct if there are any areas to clarify with the accrediting body;

- practising regular self-assessment, with reference to both personal and professional codes of conduct;

- seeking professional support in your healing practice when necessary; and

- being mindful that personal conduct is a mirror to professional practice.

3 Maintaining calmness involves:

- providing gentle lighting;

- turning off all electronic equipment;

- using music only when appropriate;

- using breathing exercises when necessary;

- developing relaxation programmes;

- using creative visualization only when appropriate; and

- cultivating a receptive attitude.

4 Wearing comfortable clothing involves:

- being aware and taking care of your appearance, especially your hands;

- having specific clothing for healing work, so that you do not take the energy from the healing circle into your everyday life;

- removing footwear when giving treatments;

- wearing clothes that are comfortable and free from restriction, so that you can move in them easily, without exposing flesh and underwear;

- wearing plain clothes if possible, in shades that are uplifting;

- limiting accessories, especially large pieces of jewellery which may come into contact with your patient; and

- carrying some form of identification, such as a badge, to verify your status as a practitioner.

5 Being a pure channel for healing involves:

- setting the intention to be a pure channel;

- taking a shower or washing both hands and feet, using unscented soaps and lotions before and after every treatment;

- asking for the mind to be cleared before the treatment begins;

- taking some conscious deep breaths to encourage a meditative state of being;

- witnessing what is taking place in the body;

- witnessing what is taking place in the mind; and

- asking to be freed from any distractions so that the healing energy may be passed freely and lightly into the patient.

6 Being prepared for a healing crisis involves:

- explaining the nature of healing and how it works from within to release energy that has been blocked or weakened;

- explaining the difference between the signs and symptoms of illness and the possibility of their being represented during the healing process;

- explaining the difference between temporary recovery, when the signs and symptoms subside, and cure, when the trauma of the illness is fully resolved;

- supporting the patient through the physical, psychological, and spiritual processes which may unfold during the healing crisis;

- explaining the support of both distant and contact healing during the processes of recovery and cure;

◆ considering the need for specific support if required from other healthcare professionals; a healing crisis may bring out areas which need the attention of other practitioners such as doctors, osteopaths or pyschotherapists; and

◆ explaining the need for time to allow both the healing crisis and the recovery period to unfold, according to the laws of nature.

7 Creating a comfortable environment involves:

◆ arranging the surroundings so that they are clean and tidy, and not holding energy released from previous treatments;

◆ using music, candles, aromatic oils and crystals only when they are appropriate for the needs of the patient, and not as an automatic ritual;

◆ providing a setting that is light and not overcrowded with objects accumulated for personal use, which may be a distraction for the patient;

◆ ensuring warmth, with blankets and extra heating if necessary, so that the patient is able to relax and respond to the healing treatment; a process that takes place when the body temperature is maintained at 37°C or 98.4°F;

◆ creating a comfortable healing space in a chair, on a couch, in a bed, or even on the floor, so that the patient feels safe and the practitioner is able to move around with ease;

◆ encouraging the patient to relax in their own time before the treatment begins; and

◆ clearing and cleaning the surroundings on a regular basis, to create an hospitable environment for patients.

Practical Exercise in Preparation for the Act of Healing

Communication: Consider what you feel to be the essence of communication.

Code of conduct: Focus on any dilemmas that you experience between personal ethics and professional behaviour.

Calmness: Reflect on how you feel when you are in the company of someone who is being peaceful.

Clothing: Observe the effect that a person's appearance makes on you when you first meet.

Channelling: Reflect on what it means to you to become a pure channel through which healing energy can be transmitted.

Crisis: Recall the most effective support that you have received during a critical period in your life.

Comfort: Remember the effect that the surroundings in surgeries and clinics have produced in you.

3.13

Contact Healing

Energy is Eternal Delight.

WILLIAM BLAKE, *THE MARRIAGE OF HEAVEN AND HELL*

When the act of healing takes place three events unfold:

1 Energy from a limitless source is mirrored through the practitioner into the patient.

2 This energy encourages the innate healing systems within the patient to work to their maximum potential.

3 During the process, energy is unblocked and freed, allowing a flow of movement to stimulate health and enhance well-being.

When taking part in the act of healing, the practitioner has three responsibilities:

1 To be a clear and receptive channel for the transmission of healing energy.

2 To be guided by the order of the treatment as it unfolds, and not to obstruct or identify with it in any way.

3 To be mindful of the patient's comfort, dignity and privacy.

Giving contact healing can be both deeply peaceful and acutely stimulating for both practitioner and patient. For practitioners, entering the state of healing consciousness may bring a stillness that allows the horizons of the present to expand. They may be aware of external surroundings, but their focus is drawn directly into the healing itself as it happens in the physical body or in the more subtle levels of energy. The practitioners' senses may become finely attuned to the changes that are taking place, allowing them to be wholly present with their patients during this time.

Receiving contact healing can also be profound, giving patients an experience of themselves which they may not have encountered before. It may take some time before a patient is ready to leave the treatment room. Drinking water, taking a few deep breaths, and imagining the feet being rooted in the earth can help ground the patient.

If a patient asks for information on what happened during a treatment, feedback needs to be given with careful consideration. The patient may be in a highly vulnerable state; giving the right amount of information in a tactful way will help them to adjust to the new arrangement of energy within. Refraining from comment, or giving too much information can be confusing and even block the outcome of the treatment. It is important to be honest and to ask for the most sensible way to express information received during the healing. Listen to any questions carefully, for within them will be contained guidance as to how to respond. Should images from the patient's energy field come into the practitioner's mind, ask for permission before imparting them. Often the answer will come through your intuitive voice and should be respected accordingly.

When the act of healing is concluded and the patient is ready to leave, the practitioner must ensure that the energy field that they have shared is separated so that they are both within their own personal fields of energy.

Practice of Contact Healing
Preparation

- ◆ Perform a simple ablution, using water if possible; otherwise, ask to be cleansed by healing energy.
- ◆ Ensure that your patient is warm and sitting in a comfortable chair.
- ◆ Take a case history if necessary.
- ◆ Answer any questions about the treatment.
- ◆ Practice some relaxation techniques if necessary.
- ◆ Explain the difference between healing through the aura or healing by touch.
- ◆ Ask for permission if you need to touch your patient.

Open up into 'Healing Mode'

Stand behind your patient.

Grounding: Ask to be present in body.

Attunement: Ask to be linked in mind to the energy of the universal healing consciousness.

Protection: Ask for protection for your own personal energy.

Permission: Ask for permission for healing to take place with your hand on the patient's shoulders.

Conduct the Act of Healing

It is possible to work through the whole energy field by scanning the energy of the chakras and meridians. Use your hands as sensors to reflect any movements that are taking place and listen to any information that arises in the process. At each stage of the scan your patient's energy will rebalance itself as much as it can under the circumstances. It is preferable to keep your hands still whilst the sensations of the patient's energy flow through them. When there are no more sensations in your hand you can then move them to the next part of the body. If you do not experience any sensations in your hands during this scan, listen to your intuitive voice, which is attuned to your patient, and follow its guidance as to when to move to the next part of the body.

Scan the chakras in the following way: starting with the crown chakra, raise your arms over the patient's head, place your hands above the chakra and sense the energy around it. Now stand at one side of the patient. Place both hands with fingers apart on either side of the chakra at the front and back of the body, but not touching it. Scan the chakras in the following order: brow, throat, heart, solar plexus, sacral and finally base.

When you have finished scanning the chakras it is now necessary to link into the meridian network.

1 Place the right hand close to the base of the spine, the palm facing upwards, and the left hand close to the back of the neck, the palm facing downwards. Sense the energy flow between the two points.

2 Move the right hand at the base of the spine up to the neck and move the left hand at the neck along to the left shoulder with both palms now facing the body. Sense the energy flow between the two points.

3   Now take your right hand and move it to the left shoulder, palm facing the body. Move your left hand to the left elbow with the palm facing it. Sense the energy flow from the shoulder to the elbow.

4   Now bring your right hand to the elbow and your left hand to the wrist, sensing the flow of energy between the two.

5   Then bring your right hand to the wrist and your left hand slightly beyond the fingers to sense the energy flow between these two points.

6   Now return your right hand to the original position in the centre of the body at the base of the spine, with the palm facing the spine this time, and bring the left hand to a point at a slight distance from the left hip, palm facing the hip. Sense the flow of energy between the spine and the hip.

7   Now bring your right hand near to the left hip and your left hand slightly in front of the left knee joint so that you can sense the energy between these two points.

8   Now bring your right hand to the back of the left ankle and your left hand to slightly away from the toes to sense the energy flow.

9   Repeat this process on the right side of the body from numbers 2 to 8.

10   When this is completed, place a hand on each foot of the patient to ground them.

11   If the treatment needs to be continued, follow your intuitive guidance as to where you need to place your hands, either on the patient with their permission or away from the body but within the field of the aura.

12   When the treatment is finished, place your hands over both feet of the patient to ground the energy.

13   Place your hands over both shoulders of your patient.

14   Close down from 'healing mode'.

Permission:	Give thanks for the healing that has taken place.
Protection:	Ask to be returned to your personal circle of energy.
Attunement:	Ask to be present in mind.
Grounding:	Ask to be present in body.

Feedback

If conversation is necessary ensure that you are in 'listening mode':

Space: Listen to your patient without interrupting.

Observation: Observe body language and respond accordingly.

Attention: Concentrate on what is being said and also what the meaning is behind the words.

Pause: Before following up on what has been said allow time for reflection. Seek to mirror, not to guide.

Figure 30: Contact healing

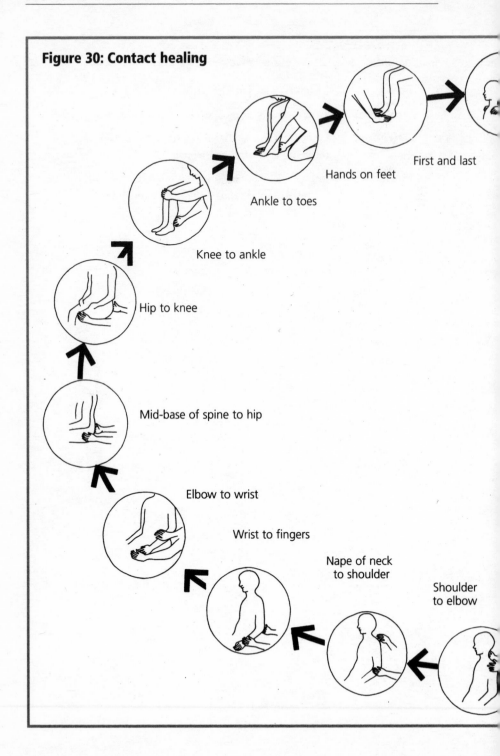

First and last

Hands on feet

Ankle to toes

Knee to ankle

Hip to knee

Mid-base of spine to hip

Elbow to wrist

Wrist to fingers

Nape of neck
to shoulder

Shoulder
to elbow

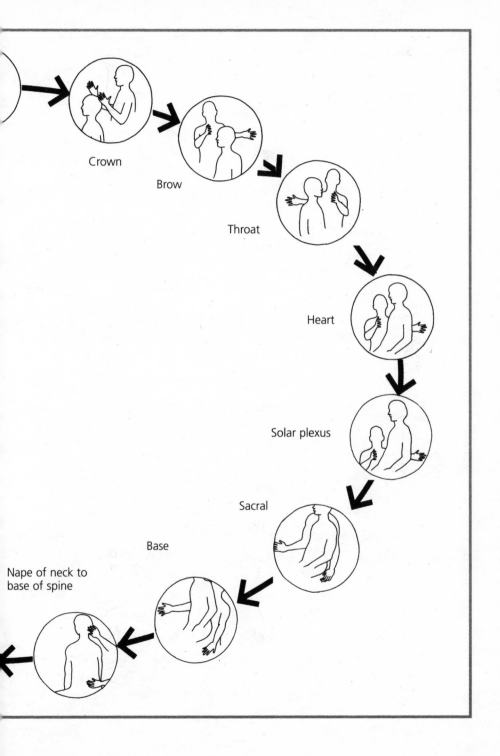

Crown

Brow

Throat

Heart

Solar plexus

Sacral

Base

Nape of neck to
base of spine

3.14

Distant Healing

Energy follows thought.

ANON

Healing can take place at any distance. It happens instantaneously when a request for healing is made, because energy follows thought. Distant healing would generally be used when there are difficulties in the patient and practitioner meeting, in cases of emergency, or at times when a full contact healing is not necessary.

It is useful to arrange a time for the healing to take place, so that the patient is ready to receive it and may gain the full benefit from it. The process of sending distant healing is similar to giving contact healing. At the agreed time the practitioner enters 'healing mode' and asks for the work to begin. When it is finished, the practitioner closes down from 'healing mode', and so concludes the treatment.

There are a number of practices which can be used, such as visualizations and dowsing with a crystal: what is important is that the practitioner follows his or her intuition to support the patient throughout the healing treatment. During this process the practitioner takes the same care as with contact healing to ensure that there is no influencing of the treatment, so that energy flows as it wills.

There is a way of acknowledging the patient at the beginning and the end of distant healing by greeting them through your heart chakra. This happens by bringing the presence of your patient into your mind's eye and looking to the reality of the whole person beyond any conditions that may define them, such as personality, lifestyle or health issues. Greeting patients in this way takes the healing energy into a far broader context, relating to their potential rather than to their limitations or problems. It puts practitioner and patient on an equal footing, uniting them in the energy of healing in complete acceptance.

Practice of Distant Healing 1
Preparation

- Arrange a time with your patient for the healing to take place.
- Perform a simple ablution, using water if possible; otherwise ask to be cleansed by healing energy.
- Bring the presence of the patient into your mind's eye and greet them through your heart chakra.

Open up into 'Healing Mode'

Grounding: Ask to be present in body.

Attunement: Ask to be linked in mind to the energy of the universal healing consciousness.

Protection: Ask for protection for your personal energy.

Permission: Ask for permission for healing to take place.

Conduct the Act of Healing

- Follow your intuitive guidance.
- Scan the energy field if necessary.
- Allow the act of healing to unfold as it wills.
- Listen to the words that you hear.
- Look at the images you see.
- Inhale any scents that you can smell.
- Absorb any flavours that you can taste.
- Feel the sensations in your body.
- What do your instincts tell you about you have experienced?
- What do you feel about it?
- What do you think about?
- Are there any images coming into view?

- What does your intuition tell you about what is happening with your patient?

- Conclude the act of healing when all these responses have been completed and your intuition tells you that the treatment is finished. Bring your patient into your mind's eye again and take your leave from your heart chakra.

Close Down

Permission: Give thanks for the healing that has taken place.

Protection: Ask to be returned to your personal circle of energy.

Attunement: Ask to be present in mind.

Grounding: Ask to be present in body.

Feedback

If the patient requests it, then do give feedback. Provide simple, truthful responses which are not coloured by your own opinions or judgements: remember, seek to mirror, not to guide.

Practice of Distant Healing 2
Preparation

- Arrange a time with your patient for the healing to take place.

- Perform a simple ablution, using water if possible; otherwise ask to be cleansed by healing energy.

- Greet your patient from your heart chakra.

Open up into 'Healing Mode'

Grounding: Ask to be present in body.

Attunement: Ask to be linked in mind to the energy of the universal healing consciousness

Protection: Ask for protection for your personal energy.

Permission: Ask for permission for healing to take place.

Conduct the Act of Healing

◆ Bring your patient into a circle of healing light.

◆ Greet your patient from the centre of your being.

◆ Ask for your patient to receive healing through the light of the universal healing consciousness.

◆ Bring your patient into your mind's eye again and take your leave from your heart chakra.

Close Down from 'Healing Mode'

Permission: Give thanks for the healing that has taken place.

Protection: Ask to be returned to your personal circle of energy.

Attunement: Ask to be present in mind.

Grounding: Ask to be present in body.

Feedback

Give feedback if asked. Provide simple, truthful responses which are not coloured by your own opinions or judgements: seek to mirror, not to guide.

3.15

Seeking Medical Help

First do no harm.

HIPPOCRATES

Working directly with energy is not a therapy but does have the potential to raise the patient's awareness of their physical, psychological and spiritual health conditions and provide the means to address them. Attending to these needs may require input from both complementary and conventional therapies, as well as from a healing practitioner.

Complementary therapies should never be used as a substitute for medical treatment. Ideally all therapies are given with the common aim of providing the correct care for the patient at the right time. They are not competing with one another if they are given in the spirit of service for the well-being of the patient. No one therapy can meet all the needs of each individual. The term 'therapist' comes from the Greek, meaning 'a person assisting in the process of healing'. Essentially the work of each therapy is assist the patient through his or her own healing process.

When seeking help for ill health it is always advisable to visit a doctor, and practitioners have a responsibility to recommend this in addition to any treatment that they may give.

Conventional treatment uses medication and surgery as its primary sources of help, and these may not only be relevant but even life-saving. We should never be embarrassed or apologetic about seeking medical help for ourselves or for others, especially the very young and the elderly. It is helpful for the patient to make a list of all symptoms, and, if these are experienced over an extended period of time, advisable to keep a diary to monitor lifestyle and the effect this may have on any medical condition.

A practitioner should encourage patients to take a real interest in their healthcare so that they can be proactive in what is required for their well-being by:

- ◆ communicating their symptoms and needs as clearly as possible,
- ◆ discussing with their doctor any effects of medical or surgical treatments,
- ◆ reading the information leaflets concerning any medication,
- ◆ exploring different choices of treatment,
- ◆ looking behind the apparent reasons for accidents and illnesses to examine their underlying causes,
- ◆ changing their doctor if they lose confidence in their treatments, and
- ◆ investigating support groups which provide information on medical conditions.

Remember that our bodies belong to us. Whatever others prescribe and advise, it is important for us to take the ultimate responsibility in our healthcare.

When to Seek Medical Help
1 Breathing Difficulties
- ◆ If they occur in a young child or a baby.
- ◆ If an asthma attack is not resolved quickly and effectively.
- ◆ If a cough lasts over 7 days and/or is associated with:
  - ◆ wheezing;
  - ◆ breathlessness;
  - ◆ yellow/green sputum.

2 Loss of Consciousness
- ◆ If it is not regained after a short period of time.

3 Bleeding

If a wound is:

- deep;
- gaping;
- contains a foreign body;
- surrounded by swelling.

If caused by:

- dog bite;
- insect stings;
- dirty instruments/objects.

4 Burns

- If the injury covers more than 1% of the body.
- If the injury destroys an entire layer of skin.

5 Bones

If there is:

- the sound of a crack;
- the site of a deformity;
- continuing pain.

6 Pain

- If it lasts longer than 24–28 hours (acute).
- If it lasts longer than 48–72 hours (chronic).
- If a severe headache is accompanied by:
  - stiff neck;
  - fever;
  - reaction to light;
  - vomiting.

7 Poisoning

If a child has consumed:

- ◆ medicine;
- ◆ chemicals;
- ◆ alcohol.

If anyone has:

- ◆ exceeded the stated dose of medicine;
- ◆ consumed an excessive amount of alcohol;
- ◆ inhaled toxic fumes;
- ◆ absorbed toxic chemicals;
- ◆ swallowed toxic chemicals;
- ◆ eaten poisonous plants;
- ◆ eaten contaminated food.

8 Infection

- ◆ If a child has a temperature over 102°F or 42°C.
- ◆ If an adult has a temperature of 104°F or 40°C.
- ◆ If a wound becomes:
  - ◆ hot, red, swollen;
  - ◆ painful/full of pus.

9 Embedded Foreign Bodies

- ◆ If any object made from materials such as glass, metal, plastic or wood penetrates the skin.

10 Heat Injuries

- ◆ When the body temperature rises above 40°C or 98.4°F.
- ◆ When the body temperature falls below 35°C or 86°F.

11 Vomiting

- ◆ If it lasts over 4–7 hours.
- ◆ If it is accompanied by diarrhoea and pain.

12 Diarrhoea

- ◆ If it lasts over 7–14 hours.
- ◆ If it is accompanied by abdominal pains.
- ◆ If it is impossible to eat or drink.

13 Status

When conditions such as asthma or epilepsy:

- ◆ persist;
- ◆ fail to respond to medication;
- ◆ get worse.

14 Instinct

- ◆ If something doesn't feel right.

A healing practitioner may be in a situation where first aid is required and it is advisable for anyone involved in healing work to take a recognized first-aid course. First-aid skills can range from putting a plaster onto a cut to giving cardiopulmonary resuscitation.

It is important to remember that all injury is accompanied by shock, and that the greater the injury, the higher the level of trauma. This condition causes the chakras to slow down or even to stop. As the chakras slow down so do all the body processes; the brain, heart and lungs draw energy for survival, depleting the other systems. If the condition of shock is not treated the healing systems cannot work to their full capacity. To remedy shock it is necessary to take the following steps:

Medical help Call for professional help if there is any doubt about the well-being of the casualty.

Rest Ease the pressure on all the body processes, especially in the brain, heart and lungs.

Warmth   Cover the casualty with blankets as the body
             temperature lowers due to loss of energy.

Reassurance Hold the casualty's hand, address the person by their
             name and answer their questions as honestly as
             possible. Don't make promises but give comfort
             through your presence.

It is important not to offer any food, in case an operation is needed which requires the casualty to have an empty stomach. Fluids may be given: usually sips of water, an ice cube to suck, or a sugary drink in the case of hypoglycaemia, when the blood-sugar levels have dropped, as in conditions such as diabetes.

The act of healing needs to be given with great caution in the treatment of shock, as the power of the energies directed towards the site of any injuries may cause them to become more pronounced. It is preferable to work through the feet to help relax the patient, as well as occasionally holding a hand or touching the body gently.

Every part of the body expresses consciousness whether or not we are aware of it. It is possible to communicate with any part of the body and to apologize to it if it has been injured. This helps to speed up recovery.

Without energy-based treatment, such as healing, shock can become trapped in the body and take months or even years to be released. The act of healing may be given at any time to treat shock. Once it is released, recovery can take place. Like childbirth, recovery takes place in three stages: the first occupying the greatest length of time, when there is little energy for anything other than the simplest tasks. The second stage becomes evident when there is more energy generated for home-based tasks but not enough to meet the needs of the outside world. The third stage, which is the briefest, becomes evident when the energy for the outside world really begins to assert itself, so that there is both stamina and enthusiasm for what lies ahead and willingness to review the illness, absorb its meaning, and consider what changes need to be made to maintain an improved state of health.

These three stages may be supported by complementary therapies: homeopathy can help to release the deep tissue bruising which accompanies physical trauma, as well as addressing psychological issues; acupuncture can free energy which may have become blocked in the meridians that supply fuel to the organs affected by the trauma of accident or illness, as well as help to relieve the impact of shock; and healing can rebalance the energy which circulates around the chakras that are affected by what has happened. Again, as in labour, there is a predictable pattern for the three stages of recovery, but no way of estimating how long a time it will take.

As everyone is unique in their responses to the trauma of accidents and illness, so they are in their ability to recover from them. Placing conditions on the time for recovery can impose a burden of obligation and guilt on those who are ill, who may then push themselves into a false sense of well-being that denies them a possibility of a full cure. All healing is dependent on letting the process evolve in its own time. Depriving it of the necessary time will prevent it from being able to do its work properly. Healing time is a period for rest, reflection and recuperation, to be valued as much as possible and appreciated for the work that is taking place to restore us to well-being and to equip us for what lies ahead.

Healing into Life

To everything there is a season
And a time to every purpose under the heaven:
A time to be born, and a time to die.

ECCLESIASTES 3:1–2

The act of healing may be given throughout pregnancy, labour and birth, to support everyone involved. The journey from conception to birth takes around 240 days. Its conditions are profoundly affected by the attitudes and responses of both parents, as well as by genetic inheritance, physical nourishment and environmental conditions present inside and outside the womb. An embryo conceived in constriction will carry this imprint throughout its life until help is given to support its release. For example, a father who feels trapped by the prospect of parenthood may imprint an anxiety of being restricted onto his child, which could manifest in conditions such as claustrophobia. Similarly, a mother who resents the responsibilities of parenthood may imprint a hypersensitivity onto her child which can cause it difficulties in making relationships.

The child is profoundly influenced by its parents through all stages of its development and whatever happens to it during this time will affect its later life. This is why it is so necessary to provide the most hospitable and loving conditions for the development of the child in the womb. There are no rigid rules to provide the framework for a satisfactory pregnancy, labour and birth. It is certainly better, whenever possible, to consider one's motives before becoming pregnant, to follow recommendations that maintain the healthy environment of the womb, and to seek help whenever it becomes necessary.

Pregnancy is an intensely demanding experience. Not only does it increase the mother's body mass but it also affects her thoughts and feelings, which can have an effect on her child. If help, including healing, is sought during pregnancy, it should never be seen as a substitute for medical supervision but as complementary to the other support services. For healing practitioners the child is as much a patient as the mother, and their work is to meet both in the present moment and to be with them throughout the treatment. Healing relates to the child in all its potential, not just to its particular stage of development. From this perspective the child also is actively engaged in coming into the world and may be seen to have its own work to accomplish in conjunction with that of the mother.

The mother's emotions are often intensified and may also be in conflict with one another. Healing during the pregnancy can help her come to terms with whatever she may be feeling during the various stages. It can also address diffi-culties encountered in previous pregnancies so that they may be resolved, allowing the current pregnancy to progress with more ease.

It is of great benefit to both patients if the healing practitioner has had some experience of pregnancy and childbirth, either personally or professionally. Empathy encourages understanding and this in turn inspires trust, all of which help to promote a productive relationship between practitioner and patient.

Healing may encourage both stamina and stability for mother and child throughout all the stages of pregnancy and birth. During and after the birth it may help to reduce the effects of trauma for both the mother and the child. The healing practitioner takes the lead from the patient, working within the intimate circle of mother and child, following their needs as they make themselves known. Although quietly and discreetly undertaken, the gentleness of such an approach may be contagious in both the labour suite and the delivery room or in the home, encouraging everyone to work towards the achievement of a good birth.

Figure 31: Energy from conception to birth

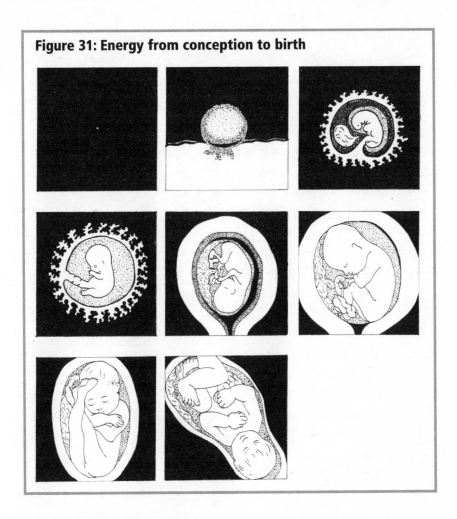

The Three Threes of Pregnancy

Weeks 1–12: Development of the form of the foetus.

Development of the placenta and umbilical cord.

Production of amnion to protect the foetus.

Weeks 12–24: The foetus embeds or 'nests' in the womb.

The foetus moves or 'quickens' in the womb.

Further growth and development by the foetus.

Weeks 24–40: The foetus takes on its own legal identity.

Chances of survival out of the womb increase.

The foetus continues to grow and develop.

The Three Signs of Labour

'Show': Release of plug of mucus which keeps closed the neck of the womb.

Waters break: Release of the amniotic fluid which cushions and protects the foetus.

Contractions: Establishment of regular abdominal muscular movement at reducing intervals of 20 minutes to 1 minute as labour escalates.

The Three Stages of Delivery

1   Opening of the cervix to approximately 10cm to allow the baby a clear passage through the birth canal.

2   'Bearing down' – the pushing movement which directs the baby down the birth canal.

3   Expulsion of the placenta and the umbilical cord from the womb.

3.17

Healing for Children

Suffer the little children and forbid them
not to come unto me; for of such is the
Kingdom of Heaven.

MATTHEW 19:14

In their early years, children are close to their origin and direct in their relationships with others. They are often drawn instinctively to people engaged in healing work, and to receiving healing energy without hindrance. One example of this is when a practitioner visits a parent to give a home treatment and the child wishes to receive healing as well. Children have a strong connection to their bodies and if given healing will absorb it enthusiastically, taking in what is necessary and recognizing when they have received enough.

The alleviation of symptoms and even full recovery may be seen quickly with them. Their body mass is smaller, the repairs more swiftly effected, and the pleasure in witnessing their recovery is heartening to family, carers and practitioners alike. Once familiar with healing, children are quick to recognize when they need it. The more they are encouraged and allowed to make their own decisions in arranging appointments, the more in touch they will become with their own needs. This will help the child to remain connected to its sense of well-being, to recognize it, and to take an increasing responsibility for maintaining it.

When working with children it is rarely possible to go through a full body scan as generally they cannot remain in one position for the length of time involved. Healing is given in a relaxed setting usually with no formal structure.

This may involve the child holding the practitioner's hand whilst sitting on a parent's lap and perhaps holding a favourite toy. Healing should never be given without the parent's permission and with the parent present if that is the child's wish. As children grow older, particularly in the teenage years, they may prefer to receive healing on their own. In this situation it may help for the parent to be present before the healing takes place and for them to return when it is completed, so that they are not excluded from the proceedings, but still respect their child's need for privacy.

Healing can be of great benefit for children who are undergoing medical treatment or who are terminally ill, giving relief from pain and helping to reduce the strong side-effects of medication such as chemotherapy. Practitioners working with children in hospital always need the agreement of the medical staff concerned as well as that of the parents.

In later years, children may become distanced from their authentic nature and less direct in their relationship with others. This connection is never lost, however, merely covered over by layers of habit as they grow older. These layers can be uncovered during the act of healing to enable the child to reconnect to its original sense of self, from which it draws solace and strength.

Childhood is a time of continual change and growth, with many adjustments that need to be made: in school, in friendships and in family life. These bring their own challenges, some of which can be stressful. Throughout childhood children can benefit from regular healing, whether or not they are ill, to help them meet these continuing demands.

3.18

Healing into Death

Everyone dies, but no one is dead.

TIBETAN SAYING

The care of the dying is as important as that of the living. The act of healing can support this care by helping the patient to accept what is happening and to prepare for their death. It can encourage them to find a perspective which is expansive, being grateful for what has been given and being open to what lies ahead. For many patients this can be a freeing process which allows them to face death with confidence.

Healing treatments can help to alleviate physical symptoms up to the point of death. When treating a patient who is dying there is no formal structure required, but rather the practitioner works through their intuition either holding the patient's hand or by working through the aura.

When working with the dying it is important for healing practitioners to look at their own reactions towards dying and death. The more we face issues relating to our own mortality, such as our ultimate powerlessness over death itself, the more we are able to support others through their passage from this world. This can help us develop sympathy, empathy and compassion towards those with whom we are working. Sympathy connects to the problem and empathy to the person. Compassion acknowledges both, but is not attached to either of them. It appears through a unified perspective which seeks only the best arrangement, whatever the circumstances.

Consciousness is not defined or limited by the decay of the physical form. If the patient is not conscious it is still possible to communicate by asking to be attuned to them at a deeper level of consciousness, which is not restricted by the conditions of the body. This can be referred to as 'the higher self'; it is not fixed by place or time because it reflects unconditioned being. During this time the practitioner should be aware of any thoughts or images that appear through the intuitive mind, be receptive to them without any interference and be willing to enter into any dialogue that needs to take place.

It may be distressing to witness the change in appearance of someone who is dying. Whatever changes are taking place on the exterior however, the interior nature of the patient remains intact. In essence, it is still the same being to whom we relate.

The healing practitioner may act as a midwife in directing the patient towards a 'good' death. With no future to plan, the present becomes increasingly important for the patient. The quality of every moment can take on a new intensity and it is here that the healing process may be of great value, in easing physical pain and feelings of loneliness, and in strengthening acceptance of oncoming death. It is important to remember the guidelines which apply in all healing practice: to be present without seeking to influence the outcome.

By investigating the stages of grief which the patient may go through at the prospect of leaving their life in this world, the practitioner is better prepared to help them. The usual stages of grief are:

Denial	('This isn't happening to me') may come from the shock that is experienced, especially at the news of sudden illness or death. This shock can create a numbness in the energy field, which gradually dissolves, allowing the news to filter through in acceptable amounts.
Anger	('How could this happen to me?') may come from the frustration of being denied a future in this life. Death after all is the ultimate arbiter over which we have no control. Anger carries a formidable energy which can be redirected into a realistic acceptance of what is happening.
Negotiation	('If I change my ways, this won't happen to me') may be an attempt to negotiate with the threat of death, by altering our outlook and behaviour. Negotiation is partial and operates at the level of cause and effect,

addressing some of the details rather than looking at the reality of the whole situation.

Depression   ('There is no meaning in what is happening to me') may emerge when the awareness of the futility of negotiating with death arises. This can be a flattening of the senses and faculties into the helplessness of desperation.

Acceptance   At the lowest ebb, resistance may dissolve into acceptance – 'this is what is happening to me' – when all of the stages have been worked through. This can also happen instantaneously, if a healing grace dissolves all difficulties and distress.

The grieving process of those who mourn a death may follow a similar pattern to those who are dying. For some, grief will be briefly felt and then released, but for others it may be delayed for months or even years, whilst there are those who may carry it for the rest of their lives.

It is important to remember that grief is for ourselves, and not for the person who has died. Grief is a natural and necessary process through which those who are mourning come to terms with death. There is no antidote except to go through it, allowing it to surface in its own time in order for memories to be encountered, apologies to be made, lessons to be learned, and finally for the grief itself to be released, so that the person who has been grieving is free to move forward.

If this process is suppressed or only partially completed then there cannot be a full resolution for those who are left behind. This can cause energy to become blocked which not only inhibits a person's potential, but can also cause physical and psychological health problems. In these circumstances the act of healing may help to release grief, however long it has been suppressed. The grief will be released according to the readiness of the patient so that they are not over-whelmed by it, but are able to allow its natural completion.

It is through experiences such as death and grief that we can open up more immediately to life and come to terms with the realization that death is a natural part of life and not an ending in itself.

Healing the Land

The land is our foundation: it blesses us with
the fruits of the earth and it behoves us to bless
it in return with gratitude for all that it yields.

ANON

There is no life without energy, whether it manifests itself in people, nature or places. As the energy of consciousness makes its journey through light, colour and sound into form it has an innate capacity to adjust and adapt to its surroundings. There are appointed pathways for the flow of energy in the land as there are in the human body.

The energy of the land circulates through chakras and travels along meridians, as it does in every form of life. These channels are referred to as ley lines and contain junction points where energy may be released or rebalanced. Many ancient monuments and places of worship are positioned on ley lines – indicating that they have been recognized and used for centuries. Their use in modern times, in land management and building projects, would allow energy to flow clearly and enterprises to prosper, because they would follow the innate intelligence of the natural order.

When there is an accumulation of negative energy in such areas as battle sites, places of execution or persecution, its effects may become apparent in the atmosphere of the place. This can also be seen when houses are built on such land and can manifest in physical or psychological illnesses, especially when they appear in clusters, and also in accidents when there are a series of them. This can be likened to ill health in a person. Negative energy, which creates a blockage in the flow, can also accumulate for other reasons such as interference with the land and more recently the siting of power cables and transmitting stations.

When the land is sick it needs to be healed: firstly by asking to be attuned to its energy, secondly by witnessing the movements of energies as they arise, and thirdly by passing on the relevant information to the people who work on it. There are many ways of healing the land, which include methods such as dowsing with rods or crystals and there are practitioners who specialize in the release of geopathic stress and feng shui consultants who are sensitive to the flow of energy in relation to the positioning of buildings and the placement of objects within them. Without linking to the fundamental source of the problem any help may bring only temporary relief rather than a permanent solution.

Working with the land uses energy in a different way from working with people. Whereas in the latter energy passes through one body into another, in clearing the land the practitioner has no physical template through which to work, but only the elements of nature, which have a power to react in a way that is infinitely stronger than that of the human form. Although the principle of healing is the same in the request to be a clear channel through which blocked energy may be released, the practice is different in that the practitioner's own energy can become much more affected because of the strength of the blockages that have accrued. Practitioners should approach this practice with caution and care. As in every other form of healing, this way of working requires education, from the experience of others who work with energy in this way, by learning about the land itself and by asking for permission from it before any healing work takes place. If there is no permission, as received through the intuitive voice, then it is necessary to ask that the land is given a blessing, so that healing can take place in the future when the time and conditions are right.

Practical Exercise: Healing the Land

For contact healing visit the area, or for distant healing use a map. Use any implements such as dowsing twigs or crystals if necessary, to help stimulate or disperse any stagnant energy.

Go into 'healing mode' before beginning the work.

◆ Grounding – ask to be fully earthed in your body.

- Attunement – ask to be attuned to the energy of the land.
- Protection – ask for protection for your own personal energy.
- Permission – ask for permission from the owner and then from the land itself for the work to take place.
- Observe any impressions and listen for any information during the healing.
- Allow the work to follow its own natural order.

Close down from 'healing mode' when the work has been completed.

- Permission – give thanks for the permission which was given and for the work that has taken place.
- Protection – ask to be returned to your own circle of energy.
- Attunement – ask to be returned to your normal state of consciousness.
- Grounding – check that you feel fully earthed in your body.
- Pass on any relevant information to the owners of the land.

3.20

Healing Places

The heavens themselves, the planets and this centre
Observe degree, priority and place.

WILLIAM SHAKESPEARE, *TROILUS AND CRESSIDA*

Traditionally, the migrating soul transits to the next plane of existence 40 days after death, an occasion which is marked in some traditions by a celebration of remembrance. There are, however, those who may not make this journey, because they are not ready to leave this world. Their presence remains in the place where they lived or died, or in a setting that was dear to them. The atmosphere in battle grounds, in areas where there were religious persecutions or scenes of mass destruction can still bear witness to these events, sometimes creating a powerful sensation of eerie stillness. Some of those who have left their physical body may still remain in spirit with their loved ones, causing people to say that the person whom they have lost is always with them.

When it is time for a presence that is in limbo, neither fully here in this world nor in there in the next one, to move on, it draws attention to its existence through the atmosphere in the rooms where it once lived, or even died. These may now feel cold and unwelcoming, resistant to all forms of heating. This can affect the current occupants of the building. They may feel uncomfortable in their surroundings, unable to settle in certain rooms and wanting to get away as often as possible. In some situations they may also become increasingly troubled by disturbing thoughts or dreams and even by recurring illnesses and misfortunes. These presences can draw energy from them to remain nourished and store it in the corners of the rooms where they often locate themselves.

Once it is clear that there are such presences, there is an opportunity for them to be released from this world so that they may make their transition into the next level of existence. This work can be carried out through the act of healing which allows communication to take place with them through attunement by the practitioner. It may be carried out on the site itself or through distant healing, using a floor plan of the space to be cleared. A crystal can be used to dowse the location of the presence and prayers or mantras spoken aloud to guide them on their way. Not only may it be more convenient to work away from the location, but it is also easier to maintain the protection required for such a powerful process.

When practising in the setting itself, it is necessary to go into 'healing mode' on entering and not to close down until leaving. Afterwards, the practitioner should always shower and change their clothing so that no traces of the work remain on them.

Working with other practitioners can be of great help. In the same way that some births require a medical team, so certain transitions after death benefit from group work to effect a safe passage from this world.

There is a distinction between those who have been unable, for whatever reason, to move on and presences which are actually malevolent in intention and behaviour. These can react very strongly to any attempt to dislodge them. Traditionally this work was often carried out by priests or religious leaders who were trained in the skills of exorcism. In general it is better to gain some experience in healing work before engaging in this area. It is never recommended that inexperienced practitioners become involved directly in clearing buildings where hostile energies are present. In these circumstances it is preferable to work with a group of practitioners from a floor plan, and initially to remain off site.

Not only can the work of healing places clear buildings of trapped or even unwelcome energies, but it is also a service to those indiscernible beings themselves, whatever the circumstances that led to their physical death, allowing them to move forward.

Working with indiscernible beings also uses energy in a different way from contact healing because the practitioner is not merely a clear channel for the flow of energy to pass through but also a support, rather like a midwife who assists at birth, in the safe delivery of the being to the next plane of existence. When working in this way, before instigating any healing process it is essential to ask for permission from the being itself through attunement to its 'higher self' rather than its present expression. If permission is refused the work should not take place, as it would only create disruption for everyone involved, since it is violating the natural order that is organic within every being. It is possible, however, to ask that the universal flow of love encompass the being so that help may be given when appropriate.

If permission to proceed with the work is given then the being is ready to make its transition from this world to the next one in a similar way to a baby as it prepares for its departure from the womb into this existence.

Practical Exercise: Healing Places

When clearing energy from buildings, go into 'healing mode' on entering the building or when opening up a floor plan if working from a distance.

- ◆ Prepare a bowl of 'sweet water', which contains spring or boiled water with some sugar dissolved in it, to be used at the end of the treatment.

- ◆ To dowse, take a crystal suspended on a thread. Go into the corner of each room and hold it up in front of you. If there is stagnant energy or a presence, the crystal will begin to move, usually in a circle.

- ◆ If a presence is located during the dowsing, greet it and then ask it for permission to be sent to the light.

- ◆ If permission is not granted, ask that the universal flow of love embraces it.

- ◆ If permission is given, follow your intuitive guidance as to which prayers, mantras or readings are appropriate to be spoken or sung aloud to encourage the presence to leave. You may also use the sounds of the chakras or meridians to assist this work.

- ◆ Again, follow your intuitive guidance as to when the presence has departed. If a presence is reluctant to leave, because the attachment has become so strong, it may be necessary to command it to go in a strong voice.

- ◆ When all the rooms have been cleared, walk through them again with the bowl of sweet water sprinkling it in all the corners and in the centre of each room.

- If any rooms have contained presences or negative energy, leave them empty for as long as possible and open any windows to allow the space to be refreshed.

- Once you have left the building or worked your way through the floor plan, close down from 'healing mode'.

- Wash the crystals or anything else that you have used for dowsing.

- Take a shower and change your clothing when you have finished.

- Destroy, preferably by burning, any floor plans that you have used, so that no connection to the presence of the negative energy remains.

When energy becomes trapped in any place, such as in our homes or where we study or work, through an accumulation of possessions or a lack of order and cleanliness, it can influence our well-being, making it more difficult for us to function effectively. There are seven guidelines which may help to prevent energy from becoming trapped and enabling it to flow more freely, creating an atmosphere of lightness and space.

1   Keep all the corners of rooms free from heavy pieces of furniture so that the energy can circulate around the room. Standard lamps, plants and ornaments can soften the sharp angles of a corner and can be easily moved for cleaning purposes. Placing copper coins in each corner of the room can also help to earth any negative energy, as can crystals, provided that they are both cleansed on a regular basis.

2   Implement a regular cleaning process for all the rooms in a home, starting from the top of the house and working downwards to ensure that energy does not become stagnant in any area.

3   Place all electronic equipment near windows which can be opened and put crystals on or close by to help reduce any harmful effects.

4   Do not have mirrors facing one another or facing windows. Too much reflected light can cause energy to be dispersed and may create an atmosphere that feels very ungrounded.

5   Keep the doors to all lavatories shut and the lids down, to prevent stale energy from waste products permeating the atmosphere in the rest of the house.

6   Arrange to have the energy cleared in your home whenever you feel it is necessary. This can be helpful after any time of crisis, such as an

accident or an illness or during any situations that have resulted in long-term stress.

7 Arrange for the energy to be cleared whenever you move into a new home, so that all the traces of the previous occupants are removed, thus preventing you from absorbing any of their energy.

Although the owner of a home may clear the energy in their own property, it is preferable to ask somebody else to carry out the work because they are less involved and can bring another perspective into the clearing work.

3.21

Healing with Animals

If you have men who will exclude any of God's
creatures from the shelter of compassion and
pity, you will have men who will deal likewise
with their fellow men.

ST FRANCIS OF ASSISI

Animals are no different from us in their elemental composition of air, water, fire
and earth, which generate blood, phlegm and yellow and black bile. The
interplay amongst these elements and fluids is controlled by the temperatures of
cold, wet, hot and dry, which produce the sanguine, phlegmatic, choleric and
melancholic temperaments.

Although animals, like their human counterparts, are characterized by a
specific temperament, the other temperaments also play a part in their constitution. All creatures have an innate intelligence, blown through the air and
carried by the blood, warmed by fire and grounded in the earth, which guides
them in their growth, development, maturity and decay.

Animals can experience a similar range of feelings to human beings,
sensing and exhibiting emotions such as fear, grief, anxiety and joy through
the element of water with an immediacy and intensity which humans may at
times suppress. Not only have they been programmed with all the resources
they need to sense danger and the skills to respond to it through the element
of fire, but also with the aptitude which enables them to find new territories in
which to establish a fresh base, through the element of air. They seek solitude

through the element of earth when it is necessary to retreat, to recover when injured or to prepare for death.

They are elemental creatures guided naturally by the light of the day and the dark of the night so that their biorhythms are in accord with the rising and setting of the sun and the phases of the moon.

It is because we are all composed of energy, albeit in configurations which are unique to each species, that humans are able to attune to the energy of animals. Animals are naturally receptive to the consciousness of healing energy when it is necessary, and do not resist it in any way, but draw on it in waves, until the healing is completed. The same principles apply to working with animals as with people and places:

- Always wait to be asked, either by the owner or by attuning to the animal's energy and witnessing its requirements.

- Confirm whether or not the animal is under medical care. If this is the case, the veterinary surgeon needs to be informed and agreement given for contact healing. This establishes the treatment in a professional context, where health practitioners do not take responsibility for patients in the care of others without their approval.

- Discuss the law of cure of the healing crisis with the animal's owner so that they are aware that a re-presentation of symptoms may occur as part of the natural process of recovery. If this happens it may be necessary to provide further contact or distant healing.

- Remember to open up into 'healing mode' prior to treatment and to close down from it at its conclusion. The energy emanating from animals may be extremely powerful, whatever their size, and should not be absorbed in any way by the practitioner.

- Encourage feedback but do not initiate it. Answer any questions as clearly as you can, but be careful of offering unsolicited advice.

Evaluate the situation if the treatments continue beyond a certain number, for example after six or seven, to ascertain whether healing is the best form of care for the animal. More input may be required in the subtle bodies, such as acupuncture for the meridians or homeopathy for the vital force, or in the physical body, with medication or surgery.

Consider personal safety, especially when treating large or potentially dangerous animals. Although treatments encourage the animal's energy field to become more relaxed, the practitioner may still be caught unawares, and require healing themselves!

In treating animals it is necessary for practitioners to accord them the same considerations that would be given to a human being. The essential integrity and dignity of the animal should be respected and the practitioner should relate to it not through its illness, but through its potential for wholeness where healing finds its perfect place.

Practical Exercise: Healing with Animals

Arrange with the owner for the timing for contact or distant healing to take place.

- ◆ Go into 'healing mode' as soon as you meet the animal.
- ◆ Maintain a gentle, unobtrusive manner with the animal.
- ◆ Be open to any images, thoughts or feelings that appear in the animal's energy field.
- ◆ Make notes if necessary so that you can give accurate information to the owner.
- ◆ Check on the animal's condition before you leave.
- ◆ Close down from 'healing mode' when you leave the animal.
- ◆ Spend time with the owner if necessary to discuss any issues relating to the animal's health that have emerged during the healing.

3.22

Healing Groups

Life is a mirror and we find only ourselves
reflected in our associates.

FLORENCE SCOVEL-SHINN

Healing groups generally come into being through the work of a small group of practitioners and may operate in a setting where members of the public are invited to attend for healing treatments. They usually grow through trainee practitioners joining the group so that they can gain practical experience in a supported situation.

To a great extent these groups are self-selecting, with members coming and going according to their personal circumstances. It is important that all members of the group become involved in its running according to their ability and experience. Although it is natural that leadership in a group will initially coalesce around a small number of people, it is better that this does not become fixed and that everyone takes part in the decision-making process.

Healing groups work at their best in an atmosphere of hospitality, where all are made welcome and encouraged to bring their own unique gifts to strengthen and maintain the team. This spirit of hospitality should extend to the patients as well, so that they are welcomed unconditionally, and not through the constrictions of illness. Everyone is gathered in healing for well-being, whether practitioner or patient.

Working in a group that treats patients on a regular basis can bring various issues to the surface such as personal relationships, healing work experience and dynamics within the structure. Healing development group work can address these in an open forum, which allows the expression of differences of opinion. Every problem has the potential to be transformed into an education in awareness which can strengthen the fabric of the group through collaborative effort. Conversely, problems hidden and unresolved weaken the cohesiveness of the group because they can be divisive causing the group to separate into factions.

Work in healing has both a private and a public face. Whilst the act of healing should remain exclusively with the practitioner and the patient, the public work of healing groups and clinics should be open to scrutiny and operate in compliance with all regulations, local or national. It carries more credibility when its members are accredited by a registered organization.

The work of healing may seem to be mysterious to members of the public who have had no personal contact with it. It is helpful to encourage anyone who wishes to find out more about the work that is taking place by visiting group sessions on an informal basis.

By following agreed guidelines in personal and professional protocol, energy healing can become better understood by the world of traditional medicine.

Guidelines for Healing Group Work

1 Clarify aims and objectives.

2 Implement protocols and procedures.

3 Observe the code of conduct of the accrediting body.

4 Follow the code of practice of the organization where the work is taking place.

5 Compile and maintain a health and safety policy.

6 Attend healing group development meetings on a regular basis.

7 Maintain a personal holistic healthcare programme.

1 Clarify Aims and Objectives

When working as a collective it is necessary to clarify the aims and objectives of the group so that it can act as one body. There is a collective strength in numbers, and when a group of people is gathered with the intention of healing it may accentuate and focus the effectiveness of its work. Aims relate to intention and objectives to implementation. The aims and objectives of a healing group may include:

◆ To maintain the primary intention in healing work, which is not a therapeutic practice but one which is given to raise physical, psychological and spiritual awareness. This may be implemented by providing a programme of continuous holistic education, to support the training given and the treatments carried out by the members of the group.

◆ To offer training in the principles and practice of healing and the language of energy. Ideally these courses should be accredited by a registered organization such as the National Federation of Spiritual Healers or other organizations which are affiliated to UK Healers, the national regulatory body.

◆ To maintain professional standards of care when working with patients by following the codes of conduct and practice as determined by the training bodies and organizations where the work is taking place.

◆ To liaise with the medical profession on a voluntary or funded basis through meetings with medical staff, hospital management and spiritual care teams to investigate the ways in which healing work can complement medical care, such as offering staff sessions on a regular basis so that they can experience healing, offering healing in hospital premises to members of the general public, organizing training programmes to explore why and how healing works and to develop proposals for permission to work with patients on the wards.

◆ To promote healing in the community by taking part in talks, workshops and exhibitions that relate to the work of healing in healthcare.

◆ To provide healing development group programmes for all the members of the group by implementing meetings on a regular basis.

◆ To offer a healing service for the practitioners in the group by arranging for suitable periods of time before or after clinic hours when healing may be given to them.

2 Implement Protocols and Procedures

Implementing protocols and procedures allows the work of healing to become both accessible in its structure and accountable in its results. Protocols relate to the presentation of the form of the group, and procedures to what evolves from it. The protocols of a healing list may include the following steps:

   i)   Take a brief case history, including details of:

- medication,
- surgery, and
- body aids.

  ii) Avoid making diagnoses.

 iii) Refrain from indiscriminate personal disclosure.

 iv) Use 'healing mode' for all treatments and related conversation:

- grounding,
- attunement,
- protection,
- permission.

  v) Exercise caution in passing on messages that come from beyond oneself.

 vi) Explain the law of cure of the healing crisis.

vii) Store all records in a safe place.

i) Take a brief case history

When giving healing to patients, in general it is necessary to take a simple case history before beginning the treatment. It can draw to attention any conditions that require special care, such as anything involving the area between the head and the neck, where three chakras, the crown, the brow and the throat are circling in close proximity to one another. The energies in the head and neck are finely balanced and require sensitive handling. In conditions like cancers affecting the head and throat, strokes, epilepsy and migraines, they may be best left alone and the work conducted through the lower parts of the body.

Other conditions to record and be aware of are artificial body parts, such as dental implants, pacemakers, new joints, and transplanted body organs. In the case of the latter there may be two sets of energy in conflict with one another, since transplanted organs will carry the energy of their previous owner. Here the energy needs to be purified, released from its previous owner so that it does not engage in conflict with its new surroundings. In the spirit of energy following thought, this can take place through the act of healing, when the request is made to free the organ from its ancestral and current memories.

Patient Record Form

NAME _____

ADDRESS _____

_____

_____

TELEPHONE _____

DATE OF BIRTH _____

STATUS   Single _____ Partner _____ Married _____

Separated _____ Divorced _____ Widowed _____

Children_____ Dependants_____

STATE OF HEALTH – Have you experienced any of the following?

Major illnesses ☐

Major stresses ☐

Operations ☐

Prolonged medication(s) ☐

Complementary medicine ☐

DISCLAIMER TO BE SIGNED WHEN NECESSARY:

I hereby acknowledge that:

  – I have been advised to seek qualified medical help for myself

  – I give permission for the child _____ who is under 16 years of age to receive healing

  – I have been advised to seek qualified medical help for the child _____

Patient _____   Practitioner _____

Patient Treatment Record

Date	Observation	Treatment	Feedback

ii) Avoid making diagnoses

Healing work relates to the flow of energy through the body but not to how it manifests in illness. It is not the responsibility of the practitioner to make a diagnosis or to determine the patient's medical care in any way, but to focus on the treatment and monitor its process.

iii) Refrain from indiscriminate personal disclosure

Healing treatments belong to the patient, not to the practitioner. Personal input from the practitioner can deflect the attention away from the patient and so disrupt the healing process. Where relevant, some personal disclosure from the practitioner may deepen understanding, but it is preferable to allow the patient the time and space to dwell on the details of their own life.

iv) Use 'healing mode' for all treatments and related conversation

This process of grounding, attunement, protection and permission (GAPP) allows access to the energy of the universal healing consciousness which is necessary during every treatment and also in the conversation that may follow from it.

v) Exercise caution in passing on 'messages'

Healing treatments are best kept as grounded as possible. When taking part in the act of healing, both practitioner and patient may have experiences that do not relate to daily life. Passing on 'messages' which come through the intuitive mind can be bewildering, upsetting and sometimes threatening to a patient. Any information received should be checked with great care to see whether it is to remain private or to be passed on to the patient. If it is to be discussed with the patient it will need to be expressed with words that are acceptable to them. For example, a practitioner may receive an actual message which is helpful for the patient. However, when introducing this in any discussion after the treatment the practitioner would not necessarily refer to it as a 'message', but rather introduce the content as a question or a comment.

The energies required for psychic work are different from those used for healing. In psychic work there is a two-way flow in which the practitioner acts as a filter, choosing how much information is to be passed on and returning the rest to its source. In healing work there is a one-way flow in which the practitioner acts as a vessel for energy to flow into the patient.

Mixing the two ways of working can create confusion in the psyche of the practitioner as they both require acute and specific levels of concentration. Developing skills in any area of life requires time and application. In this instant it is preferable to make a conscious choice between the two and to follow the one that validates personal integrity.

vi) Explain the law of cure of the healing crisis

It is helpful for patients receiving healing to understand the law of cure of the healing crisis, in which a decline in energy may precede recovery. Prior to the treatment the patient may have experienced symptoms of physical traumas, psychological episodes, and spiritual crises. During or after the treatment these symptoms may be revisited, causing distress for a brief period of time before the balance of health is restored.

vii) Store records in a safe place

It is helpful to keep a record of all healing treatments that are given on a private basis and necessary for those given on a professional one. Storing all records of treatments securely in a locked box or filing cabinet and all computer-written notes according to any relevant data protection requirement helps to preserve the confidential nature of the relationship between practitioner and patient. All introduction records should be signed by the patients; a second signature may be necessary to give permission for notes to be stored on computer and to be included in a database. This guarantees that, in the UK for example, there will be no selling of names to other organizations.

There are seven basic reasons for keeping records of healing treatments, which are:

- ◆ to recall the treatment so that there is the opportunity to reflect on what has taken place;

- ◆ to record essential, factual details about the patient which will need to be passed on should there be a change of practitioner;

- ◆ to monitor the progress of healing treatments for the patient, the practitioner and, if required, for any future legal representation should issues relating to malpractice occur;

- ◆ to formalize the practitioner-patient relationship so that family or friendship connections do not confuse it;

- to respect both the informal rule of confidentiality and the formal laws of data protection;
- to follow the governing laws of the country regarding the treatment of children and animals;
- to maintain the health and safety of both the practitioner and patient, whether in a public or a private place, with regard to local regulations. This includes passing on information to the relevant authorities about any potential or actual risks which come to notice.

When making home visits it is advisable to work in pairs if the patient is a stranger and to leave details with someone of the time of the treatment and the name, address and telephone number of the patient.

Outdated notes should preferably be shredded to preserve the privacy of the patient-practitioner relationship.

Describing the procedure which applies to every patient who is treated by a member of a healing group unifies the proceedings, so that everyone is treated in a similar way. Although every treatment evolves according to its specific arrangement, it comes under an order which is accepted by all the practitioners. Procedures may include:

- greeting the patient in a friendly manner;
- noting the time of their arrival;
- filling in a patient treatment record card;
- escorting them to the waiting area;
- indicating the toilet facilities;
- indicating the emergency exits in case of fire;
- offering drinks such as water, juice, tea or coffee;
- introducing the healing practitioner;
- following the order of arrivals in allocating treatments;
- escorting the patient into the treatment area;
- taking a brief case history;
- conducting the healing treatment;
- escorting the patient back to the waiting area;

- offering water to drink to encourage grounding;

- taking the patient to a quiet area, if there is need for further conversation;

- making another appointment if it is appropriate;

- discussing the possibility of distant healing as a follow up to the current treatment;

- discussing a home visit if it is necessary;

- checking that the patient feels grounded and ready to leave;

- accepting and recording a donation if it is made;

- bidding the patient goodbye;

- completing the treatment record card and storing it securely;

- debriefing with the group leader if information shows that a patient is at risk, to explore what action needs to be taken.

3 Observe the Code of Conduct of the Accrediting Body

Observing the relevant code of conduct of the training organization to which all the practitioners should belong brings them into alignment with one another in relation to professional standards of practice. It may also be a legal obligation in order to meet the insurance requirements which have to be taken out as a protection for the patient and also against any possibility of litigation. All patients have legal rights, which are explained in the code of conduct of the accrediting body, and practitioners are entrusted with the responsibility for upholding them. Healing work, like any other form of healthcare, operates within the legal framework of the country concerned and it is important for prac-titioners to comply with all the relevant regulations.

4 Follow the Code of Practice of the Organization where the Work is Taking Place

Following the code of practice of the host organization where the healing group operates is also necessary both personally and professionally. The practi-tioners are guests who need to be aware of the courtesies of hospitality, such as not rearranging their surroundings, maintaining them with care and not leaving behind any traces of their activities when they depart.

5 Compile and Maintain a Health and Safety Policy

It is necessary to formulate and maintain a health and safety policy which is in accord with both the accrediting body of the practitioners and with the host organization such as the National Health Service, whose facilities are being used. A health and safety policy protects the well-being of both practitioners and patients and prepares a setting in which there is minimal risk of harm. It is necessary to undertake a basic audit of the potential risks and the known hazards in the environment where healing work is taking place. This may be formulated by:

- listing the activities that take place during the time when the group meets;
- identifying any potential danger in any of these activities;
- identifying any people who may be at risk, such as people in wheelchairs or those who are suffering serious illnesses;
- assessing the possibility of any injuries that could occur;
- establishing cautionary measures to prevent such injuries from taking place;
- evaluating existing measures to affirm their effectiveness;
- providing training programmes to increase awareness of potential danger.

It is also helpful for practitioners to have a working knowledge of first aid so that they can respond quickly and effectively if a patient becomes unwell. Should this happen it is necessary to bring it to the attention of the rest of the group for future reference.

Health and safety checklist

Data	Practitioner	Patient	Contact
Name			
Address			
Telephone numbers			

Treatment details

Date		Time	
Treatment			

Environment outside the home

Safe weather	Clear directions	
Adequate parking	Safe pathways	
Adequate lighting	Access to home is well lit	

Environment inside the home

Floors	Lighting	
Furniture	Ventilation	
Hygiene/washing facilities	Household pets	

Assessment of risks

Patient's behaviour

Smoking

Medications

Substance abuse

Harmful weapons

Assessment outcome

Hazards

Safety

Signature: Date:

6 Attending Healing Group Development Meetings on a Regular Basis

Attending group development meetings on a regular basis encourages ongoing education in the practice of healing. Issues addressed may include:

- how the group is administered;

- how to implement projects to make the work more widely known;

- when to provide role-play practice, especially in conversation skills, to draw out the difference between advising and supporting patients through their difficulties;

- how to maintain a holistic approach when working with patients, so that they are not defined by their illness, but rather by their potential for well-being;

- how to encourage everyone to speak without interruption, so that voices are heard one at a time;

- how to cultivate ideas within the group so that they inspire its members to take healing work forward through collaborative effort;

- how to co-ordinate the group to establish effective working relationships in which everyone feels valued for their contribution and their commitment to the work of healing.

Healing development group record

Session: _____ Date: _____

Attending:

Agenda:

Action:

Quote of the session:

Book of the session:

Date of next meeting:

7 Maintain a Personal Holistic Healthcare Programme

Maintaining a personal healthcare programme is as essential for people working in healing as it is in all other caring disciplines. This work can have a profound effect on the energy field of the practitioner as well as that of the patient. It may cause changes to occur which themselves require treatment through healing, complementary therapies or allopathic medicine. It is vital for practitioners to attend to their own well-being so that they become a clear mirror for their patients. Aspects of personal healthcare in relation to healing work include:

- ◆ checking one's own motives regularly in undertaking healing work;
- ◆ refraining from giving healing treatments when feeling physically ill or mentally stressed;
- ◆ leaving enough space between treatments to become refreshed before the next patient arrives;
- ◆ finding a balance between giving healing treatments and engaging in other forms of healthcare work;
- ◆ ensuring there is not an excessive involvement with a patient's condition;
- ◆ arranging healing treatments for oneself as necessary;
- ◆ remaining grounded in everyday life through activities which involve some physical work.

As healing work evolves continually, so does a healthy group. It needs to be able to learn from any problems that have arisen in the past, make any necessary changes and ensure that the service it provides meets the needs of the patients.

3.23

Healing in Hospitals

The very first requirement in a hospital
is that it should do the sick no harm.

FLORENCE NIGHTINGALE

Hospital work and healing are both dedicated to healthcare but the routes that are taken are different: hospitals offer surgical and medical treatments for specific conditions, whereas healing relates to the health of the whole person. Allowing healing practitioners to complement medical treatment by working with patients can provide sensitive and effective support during times of crisis and periods of recovery.

Healing practitioners working in hospitals need to observe the codes of ethics and conduct which apply to all the other staff. As well as being accredited by registered organizations, they need to undertake formal training in working with energy and have some knowledge of first aid and health and safety. They must also be covered by insurance. Although gentle in touch, healing can be powerful in results and when working in groups the work needs to be supervised by the group leader or a designated sponsor.

When formulating a proposal for healing to be offered within a National Health Service setting there are seven aspects to be considered:

1 What are the reasons for offering the healing service?

- ◆ Increased choices for patients;
- ◆ increased relaxation;

◆ relief from pain;

◆ greater ability to respond to treatments;

◆ less need for medication;

◆ increased access to inner resources of strength and acceptance;

◆ reduced length of time spent in hospital.

2 What evidence is there of its effectiveness?

◆ Anecdotal;

◆ scientific;

◆ media coverage.

3 What systems are already in place in the NHS that already offer healing services?

◆ Hospitals;

◆ GP clinics;

◆ community services.

4 How would the system operate within the proposed setting?

◆ Liaison between healing practitioners and medical staff;

◆ allocation of practitioners to different departments.

5 What are the training, support and supervision services offered to the healing practitioners?

◆ Accredited educational courses;

◆ mentor supervision;

◆ CPD programmes;

◆ insurance requirements.

6 How will the service be funded?

◆ Is it free for all of the patients?

◆ How will the practitioners be paid?

7 How will the service be assessed for its effectiveness?

- ◆ Patient feedback forms;
- ◆ follow-up responses;
- ◆ regular meetings with the other healing practitioners;
- ◆ regular team meetings with the medical staff.

Seven reasons for bringing healing into the hospital environment are:

1 To demonstrate how energy healing can complement medical care

This can be achieved firstly by providing one or several healing practitioners who are trained and registered with an accredited organization and who are supervised by a team leader in agreement with the ward manager. Secondly, it can be achieved by keeping records of healing treatments so that their effectiveness may be evaluated regularly by the medical staff.

2 To work with the energy of the wards

In addition to working with patients, healing may be given to clear the energy in the wards. This work should be carried out through distant healing, using a floor plan of the whole department. When there are a number of ill people in a room a general atmosphere may develop through an exchange of energy in depleted or disrupted auras. The law of energy states that the weak draws from the strong; in this situation energy can be drained from those in recovery by those who are critically ill or in decline. There are also illnesses that may develop from being in hospital, as well as those that brought the patient there in the first place. Clearing sick energy from a ward is as necessary as maintaining an impeccable level of hygiene, and should be carried out on a regular basis. This work can validate itself both in the lifting of the atmosphere, so that the patients, staff and visitors feel more at ease in the surroundings, and also in improved rates of recovery and a reduction in hospital-transmitted infections.

3 To support the health of the hospital staff

Staff work programmes are often hectic and demanding. They are attending daily to people whose lives are in crisis or in great need of support in the face of chronic illness. When employees are given healthcare such as healing, which is unobtrusive and often has a calming effect, they are better prepared to care for their patients because they have attended to their own well-being.

4 To complement the work of all the staff

Allowing healing practitioners to work with patients can give staff more space to fulfil their specific tasks. Healing practitioners may have more time to spend with the patients because their work is nonspecific: its function is to be present, for as long as is necessary, until energy is flowing to its maximum potential.

5 To promote recovery

This may be particularly helpful after surgery, for the healing of wounds and for all invasive procedures such as canulation and investigative X-rays. Again, this service can only be validated by its results. All genuine healthcare, including healing, should be open to investigation: it can only benefit from the feedback that thorough research would offer it.

6 To provide help during birth and death

Although mortality rates in childbirth have been reduced greatly, every labour is accompanied by the possibility of death. During this time the act of healing can not only calm mother and child, but also reduce the birth trauma, which otherwise may only be released later in life through subtle procedures which work directly with energy, such as sacro-cranial work and healing. Conditions such as dyslexia, dyspraxia, autism and hyperactivity syndromes may all develop through lack of oxygen during labour and birth. It could be a great gift to every newborn baby to be given healing so that it may recover as fully as possible from the rigours of its birth.

Every death is a rite of passage, and needs to be honoured as such. When healing is given it may ease not only physical pain but also the psychological struggle which may come about in the wake of impending decease. It may even be sent after death to support patients in the transition from this world to the next, or to assist them in letting go of the bonds which hold them in this earthly plane of existence.

7 To liaise with patients' families during times of distress

Healing is given unconditionally in the wisdom of right timing, so that whatever needs to appear finds the place to do so. It doesn't necessarily alter what is happening, but it may help to change how people feel about it, and help them to access inner resources of resilience and fortitude.

The leader of a healing team needs to formulate two documents, one to be kept for personal reference and the other to be lodged with the ward manager. The team leader's document should include:

- aims and objectives;
- protocols and procedures;
- names, addresses, email details, land line, mobile and work telephone numbers of all the practitioners;
- qualifications;
- certificates of insurance;
- two references, one personal and one professional;
- code of conduct of the accrediting body;
- articles and general information relating to healing.

The ward manager's document should contain:

- aims and objectives;
- protocols and procedures;
- names and qualifications of healing practitioners;
- training and support services;
- code of conduct;
- articles and general information relating to healing work.

It is important to describe the order of procedure for a healing treatment, and the follow-up processes which include debriefing with team leaders and medical staff and the safekeeping of records. It is also necessary to give a full account of training programmes and continuous personal development initiatitives, to ensure that education in healing is ongoing and dynamic in response to whatever is encountered through work experience. When healing is given in a public setting, such as a hospital ward, its benefits may be contagious, affecting not only those being treated but also others in the immediate vicinity. Healing offers the most fundamental type of healthcare, supporting every therapeutic procedure, because it addresses both the general condition of the illness as well as the unique nature of the patient which is essentially unlimited in its capacity to heal itself.

Practical Exercise: Working with a Patient in a Hospital Ward

If a patient has asked you to visit them in hospital to give a healing treatment, take the following steps.

- ◆ Contact the ward manager prior to the treatment to request permission for the work to take place and make arrangements for your visit.
- ◆ Introduce yourself to the medical staff before beginning the treatment.
- ◆ Wash your hands before and after every treatment.
- ◆ Enter into 'healing mode' when you greet the patient.
- ◆ Create as much privacy as possible for your patient, screening the bed or using another room for the treatment if one is available.
- ◆ Hold your patient's hand or sit quietly by the bedside to conduct the healing.
- ◆ Follow your intuitive guidance in the order of the treatment.
- ◆ Watch carefully for any signs of distress in the patient.
- ◆ Find a member of staff if you feel concern about any change in the patient's condition.
- ◆ Take time for conversation if the patient wishes.
- ◆ Sit quietly for a while if you feel that the patient needs support.
- ◆ Close down from 'healing mode' at the end of the treatment.
- ◆ Give any appropriate feedback to the medical staff.
- ◆ Record any factual details of the treatment if required such as changes in breathing, colour, or relief from pain.
- ◆ Inform a member of staff when you leave the ward.

Practical Exercise: Clearing the Energy of a Hospital Ward

◆ Make a number of copies of a floor plan of the whole department so that this procedure can be repeated on a regular basis.

◆ Use the distant healing format with a floor plan for clearing the energy of the department.

◆ Enter into 'healing mode'.

◆ Use an implement such as a crystal suspended on a thread for dowsing the premises.

◆ On the plan place the crystal over the corner of each room and hold it still in front of you.

◆ If the crystal begins to move, say or sing appropriate prayers, mantras or readings until the movement in the crystal stops.

◆ Close down from 'healing mode' when the work has been completed.

◆ Cleanse any implements that you have used.

◆ Destroy the floor plan so that no traces of energy from the clearing remain with you.

◆ Inform the medical staff of any relevant information.

3.24

Healing and Spirituality

Without a generous heart
there can be no spiritual nature.

GAUTAMA THE BUDDHA

Healing is an expression of spirituality and proceeds from it. In healing there is lightness of touch; in spirituality, lightness of being. Through light we return to our essential nature, prior to form, sound and colour. Light illuminates life so that it may be seen everywhere. The spiritual nature seeks enlightenment where it becomes at one with itself, a clear mirror for self-reflection.

In healing there is openness of heart. In spirituality there is openness of mind, ultimately to allow consciousness to be suffused with love, the guiding force which frees us from constriction and encourages us to value life rather than to diminish or block its potential through those thoughts and actions which are constrictive in nature.

In healing there is the love of understanding; in spirituality the love of truth which awakens us to the reality of ourselves as we are now.

In healing there are no barriers in communication between practitioner and patient; in true spirituality there is no denial of any one form of belief, but an acceptance that everyone needs to discover meaning according to their own unique nature and understanding.

In healing there is an infinite source of energy; in spirituality an endless resourcefulness that nurtures the being through all the cycles of life experience. It is ever present, yet only accessed through conscious choice, which makes its gifts readily accessible.

In healing there is faith that there is such a reality as healing energy; in spirituality there is trust that there is an order and meaning to life to be discovered and followed.

In pure healing there is no attachment; the work takes place for its own sake beyond the limitations of the practitioner and patient. In spirituality there is no identification with any specific state of being. It arises through the breath, adapting to every instant. It cannot be defined by any terms, even that of being 'spiritual'; it inspires us to go on, for the love of life itself, wherever it may lead us.

3.25

Healing for the Whole Person

What is whole in a person relates to their potential and their actuality. These are not separate from one another but are different expressions of energy, the one hidden and the other revealed. The potential of a person is unconditional; it cannot be defined or measured, unlike activities in the body and responses from the mind. It can, however, be accessed by being receptive to deeper levels of consciousness, through flashes of inspiration, by learning from what has already happened in life, and in practices such as contemplation and meditation.

The work of healing relates to all the bodies of energy at every level. It goes where it is needed, moving throughout the auric bodies with inspired and intelligent ease. All the bodies are designed to function efficiently and to co-operate with one another; when any malfunction appears, repair systems come into being, restoring balance and maintaining the equilibrium within the energy fields to the best of their capacity. The repair systems are most evident in the outer fields of energy; meditation and prayer can bring healing to the inner levels of being. As the energy becomes more accessible in the mind and the body, so access to the healing systems becomes more tangible.

There are a number of energy therapies which relate directly to the movement of energy, such as acupuncture, aromatherapy and homeopathy. Healing alone acts without intermediary. It comes from the request for it, for all the bodies of energy to work to their full potential. In stimulating the energetic bodies into action it can fulfil its function, provided that there is no imposition or interference from either the healing practitioner or resistance from the patient, when the time is right.

When energy flows freely, all living beings are grounded by earthly influences and open to the heavenly spheres, moving between the two, never fixed but always fluent in the ability to draw inspiration from both of them.

With humility, life can be accepted as a gift, which cannot be conditioned by us in any way. It is given for experiencing and educating so that we may come to know ourselves. Our relationship to it can be transformed by love so that we may accept ourselves as we are in our reality, in all our weaknesses and strengths. When the healing practitioner is inspired by the love of service, the flow of healing may become unconditional in its potential, ready to respond to any request that is made for it. This is our birthright, since life is for healing, for becoming whole.

Wholeness is the potential in every moment for completion. It is complete within itself yet always carries the possibility for further unfolding. As the bounty of life is never-ending, wherever it manifests, so is the capacity for wholeness in which we may be transformed by the knowledge of love in a journey that never ends.

Index